Practical Healthcare Statistics with Examples in Python and R

Practical Healthcare Statistics with Examples in Python and R provides a clear and straightforward introduction to statistical methods in healthcare. Designed for recent graduates, new analysts, and professionals transitioning into healthcare analytics, it offers practical guidance on tackling real-world problems using statistical concepts and programming.

The book is divided into three primary sections. The first section provides an introduction to healthcare data and measures. In these chapters, readers will learn about the nuances of administrative claims and electronic health records, as well as common industry measures related to quality and efficiency of care. The second section will cover foundational techniques, such as hypothesis testing and regression analysis, as well as more advanced approaches, like generalized additive models and hierarchical models. In the last section, readers will be introduced to epidemiological techniques such as direct and indirect standardization, measures of disease frequency and association, and time-to-event analysis.

The book emphasizes interpretable methods that are both effective and easy to communicate to clinical and non-technical stakeholders. Each technique presented in the book is accompanied by statistical notation described in plain English, as well as a self-contained example implemented in both Python and R. These examples help readers connect statistical methods to real healthcare scenarios without requiring extensive programming experience. By working through these examples, readers will build technical skills and a practical understanding of how to analyze healthcare data.

These methods are not only central to improving patient care but are also adaptable to other areas within and beyond healthcare. This book is a practical resource for analysts, data scientists, health researchers, and others looking to make informed, data-driven decisions in healthcare.

Michael Korvink serves as Principal, Research and Innovation at Premier, Inc., and is a member of the graduate teaching faculty in the Public Health Sciences Department at the University of North Carolina (UNC) at Charlotte. In his current role at Premier, Michael is responsible for collaborative research across health systems, academic institutions, and government agencies. Michael has over 20 years of experience in the healthcare and pharmaceutical industry and publishes regularly on research methods related to quality, safety, and efficiency of care. Michael holds a Master of Arts from UNC Charlotte, is a professional accredited statistician (PStat) through the American Statistical Association, and is pursuing a doctorate in public health at the Medical College of Wisconsin's Institute for Health and Humanity.

Practical Healthcare Statistics with Examples in Python and R

A Guide for the Uninitiated

Michael Korvink

CRC Press
Taylor & Francis Group
Boca Raton London New York

CRC Press is an imprint of the
Taylor & Francis Group, an **informa** business

A CHAPMAN & HALL BOOK

Designed cover image: Shutterstock_1746754541

First edition published 2025
by CRC Press
2385 NW Executive Center Drive, Suite 320, Boca Raton FL 33431

and by CRC Press
4 Park Square, Milton Park, Abingdon, Oxon, OX14 4RN

CRC Press is an imprint of Taylor & Francis Group, LLC

© 2025 Michael Korvink

ISBN: 978-1-041-00423-3 (hbk)
ISBN: 978-1-041-00141-6 (pbk)
ISBN: 978-1-003-60975-9 (ebk)

DOI: 10.1201/9781003609759

Typeset in Palatino
by SPi Technologies India Pvt Ltd (Straive)

To Jen, who has shown me that the heart of healthcare lies not in statistics but compassion and dedication at the bedside. To Maddie, may you succeed in everything you seek, both on and off the mat. Keep going!

With love,
Mike

Contents

Preface

The goal of this book is simple: to help the beginner analyst approach common healthcare problems using foundational, time-tested, and interpretable statistical methods.

I write this book as a professional who has worked as a foot soldier in the healthcare and pharmaceutical industry for 20 years—with most of those years spent doing hands-on analysis. I'm currently a researcher for a large healthcare organization, where I spend most of my time implementing statistical models using patient data and mentoring others. I have published regularly during this time, using many of the techniques outlined in this book. I have also taught courses on data mining at the University of North Carolina at Charlotte, where I helped students grasp foundational statistical concepts and apply them tactically to real-world healthcare problems. I will stress, however, that this book is not academic but is designed to be a practical guide for the working professional. As such, I will avoid veering off on theoretical tangents and focus on the practical application of the methods related to specific healthcare problems. I avoid statistical jargon when possible and have attempted to explain these concepts as I would to a recently hired college graduate or intern.

I know it can be overwhelming to do statistics outside of the controlled environment in the classroom. When beginning to conduct statistics in the wild, it can feel like the formal education in the classroom is far removed from the day-to-day work conducted in the industry. I was hired at my current employer nearly 15 years ago, and my first assignment was to help translate the statistical documentation of a risk adjustment model (more about risk adjustment later) to a team of Java developers so that they could make an important update to the methodology. While I had some basic technical skills and domain knowledge at the time, having worked in pharma for five years prior, I was admittedly overwhelmed by the learning curve ahead of me.

I was provided a methodology document written by a seasoned statistician, a Harvard PhD no less, who had liberally decorated his documentation with (at the time) cryptic statistical notation. Not only was I out of my league from a statistics perspective, but I also did not have the foundational healthcare knowledge to thoroughly understand the business problem being solved. Exacerbating the issue, I struggled to translate the statistical notation to the technical implementation. I began cobbling together various resources to decipher this methodology and how it would be implemented using code. At the time, I recall saying that I wished a book existed that outlined the basic concepts of healthcare statistics and the programmatic implementation. I wanted to see the notation side by side with the code in the context of healthcare.

In a sense, this is the book I wish I had as a newcomer to the healthcare space. There are many fantastic introductory statistics books, and there are also many well-written primers on healthcare data. However, books introducing statistics in the context of the healthcare setting are scarce, and when limited to those written for a professional audience, even fewer options exist. I am hopeful that this book will be the resource that I wanted at the time for newcomers to the healthcare space.

This book is not simply an introduction to statistics presented with healthcare-related examples. In the following chapters, we'll certainly discuss foundational statistical methods, such as the hypothesis testing framework, but we will also introduce techniques that are often represented in the healthcare setting (e.g., risk adjustment, standardized ratios, survival analysis). I will not be shy about introducing more "advanced" concepts such as generalized additive, hierarchical, and zero-inflated models, as these methods overcome common problems that regularly occur within healthcare analyses. Data that is non-linear, has multiple levels, and has a high percentage of zeros are common among everyday problems. Without awareness of these methods, beginner analysts may feel that their hands can be tied—causing them to leap too quickly to less interpretable ML/AI approaches. These methods will be presented only after an overview of healthcare data sources and measures frequently used in healthcare analyses.

One might think of this book as an orientation to healthcare analyses, designed to take the reader from concept to implementation (with some admittedly bad jokes along the way). While the primary audience for this book includes beginner data analysts, data scientists, health researchers, and statisticians in the healthcare domain, I believe that the concepts discussed here will also benefit individuals in more senior roles or peripheral roles, such as business analysts, product owners, and healthcare leaders. Statistical literacy is invaluable for all professionals involved in healthcare decision-making, as it enables them to ask the right questions, interpret data-driven results, and make informed choices.

To narrow the scope of this book further, I will emphasize statistical measures and methods central to patient care and utilization. After all, the patient is at the center of all healthcare disciplines. Other aspects of healthcare, such as labor and supply chain, are important domains; however, attempting to boil the ocean by including the many facets of healthcare outside of patient care would, unfortunately, dilute the content of this book. That said, the statistical methods discussed here remain transferrable to other domains in healthcare (and outside of healthcare).

I'll stress that we will focus on interpretable methods using applied statistics. Within the healthcare space, we must have the tools to explain our findings meaningfully to our clinical stakeholders. In 2021, I collaborated with a research team of surgeons, quality administrators, and public health researchers. We employed a multivariable hierarchical logistic regression model (yes, we'll talk about this too), evaluating how various aspects of care prior to a total hip arthroplasty (THA) were associated with a patient's risk of readmission. Our work, published in the *Journal of Arthroplasty*, concluded, for example, that the use of tranexamic acid and spinal anesthesia during total hip arthroplasty is associated with reduced odds of readmission. We were able to quantify the odds with a measure of statistical significance, grounding the analysis in a reproducible framework. The use of interpretable methods in that analysis was vital to our collaboration as we were able to speak a common language throughout the process and articulate our results to the academic community using industry-accepted methods.

But Mike, isn't the field of statistics becoming antiquated with recent developments in machine learning (ML) and artificial intelligence (AI) models? The field of statistics is foundational and is the backbone of many ML/AI models, and one might argue that both ML and AI fall under the broader umbrella of statistics. Linear regression is not going anywhere soon, and I will argue that these foundational methods should first be considered before moving to more advanced ML models. I will also argue that there is a range of generalized models that sit in between the models that are commonly associated with statistics and ML that are often overlooked, especially in the field of Data Science (I am in that field, and this comment is not meant to disparage Data Scientists). Many times in my career, I have seen a new analyst quickly abandon a regression-based model for an eXtreme Gradient Boosted (XGBoost) or neural network model the moment that performance is inadequate or the regression assumptions are violated. Confession time: I, too, have been guilty of this in my early career. A generalized additive model (GAM), for example, is, in my opinion, an often-overlooked model that has the benefit of interpretability, like that of linear or logistic regression, but also gracefully handles non-linearity between the independent and dependent variables.

Another argument for interpretable methods revolves around gaining buy-in from the clinical and non-technical stakeholders. I have witnessed projects fail in a nanosecond due to analysts attempting to explain the incredible wizardry of their ensemble model to physicians, only to be received by blank stares. While your deep reinforcement learning model with gradient-based hyperparameter optimization may result in an optimal k-fold cross-validated mean squared error, it is worthless if it is never implemented to improve the quality of care and drive root cause improvement. Projects that can be explained to stakeholders are more likely to be supported by leadership and adopted by the consumers of those models.

Most problems encountered in everyday analysis can be approached with direct statistical methods. We should exhaust these options before leaping to more advanced ML/AI methods. Models such as XGBoost tree models and convolutional neural networks certainly have their place in healthcare, and I use ML in my work; however, if the goal is to explain to the Chief Nursing

Officer of a major health system the drivers behind increased central line-associated bloodstream infection (CLABSI) occurrences or interpret the relationship between age and hemorrhage risk in delivering mothers, it will be difficult to gain trust and buy-in without clearly stated interpretable results with transparency around the estimated error in the data.

It would be nearly impossible to provide an overview of healthcare, statistics, and R and Python programming from the ground up. Given that the primary audience of this book is a recent graduate or an individual transitioning into a healthcare analysis role, I will assume that the reader has taken an introductory statistics course or has a fundamental knowledge of descriptive statistics. The reader should know what a mean, median, standard deviation, and percentile are and have a working knowledge of basic data types such as discrete and continuous quantitative data and nominal and ordinal qualitative data.

I will also assume that the reader is a beginner in Python or R, at a minimum. We will not discuss setting up a development environment or using the many IDEs available. Furthermore, no crash course on Python or R programming is provided in these pages. There are many well-written resources for those beginning Python and R-based data analysis, and duplicating those efforts here would take away from the healthcare-focused analysis this book is designed to provide. Finally, this book will not discuss data "munging" or data processing to prepare analytic datasets. There are a multitude of books on data analysis using Python or R, and it is advised that readers seek those resources for foundational knowledge on data analysis.

We will use code only as a means to an end and will use the core data manipulation and statistical packages when possible. In Python, examples primarily use `pandas`, `NumPy`, `statsmodels`, `scipy.stats`, and `scikit-learn`. In R, we will use core base R functions when possible and will rely on mature, well-supported libraries when no base R support is available (e.g., `mcgv`, `lme4`, `survival`). The examples provided will be procedural (for ease of reproducibility) using arrays and data frames, and as such, we will avoid examples using object-oriented approaches.

Techniques will be demonstrated with small self-contained reproducible examples (or "reprex", as our friends at Posit say). For each coding example, I've tried to follow a consistent pattern where a small data frame of mock data is created in-line prior to the demonstration of the technique. This allows the examples to be executed without dependencies on outside datasets. There are admittedly tradeoffs with this approach, as in-line data generation limits the volume of that data and the potential sophistication of the example. That said, I prefer to work with small toy examples such as these, knowing there are some disadvantages with this approach.

While this book is designed such that each chapter builds on the chapters before it, I've tried to minimize the dependencies so that the reader can read each chapter or group of chapters in isolation. Those interested in foundational healthcare data might read Chapters 1 and 2, where an overview of healthcare data sources, standards, and industry measures are discussed. Chapters 2–5 will focus on foundational statistical methods ranging from hypothesis testing to regression analysis. Chapters 7–9 will focus on techniques common within epidemiological research, including risk standardization, measures of disease frequency and association, and time-to-event analysis (a.k.a. survival analysis).

I hope you find the information in this book useful as you embark on your career as an analyst in the healthcare field. I remained in a constant state of anxiety as I wrote this book, always worried that I was overexplaining or underexplaining a particular concept or idea. I felt guilt for excluding important topics and hesitated including others. This book is, after all, a product of my career, experiences, and education, and in this first edition, I'm sure there is room to improve. I welcome your feedback as you read this book and can be reached at mikes_stat_book@protonmail.com. I would be glad to hear what aspects of the book you enjoyed and where you believe improvement can be made. Please reach out!

Acknowledgments

I want to express my deepest gratitude to all those who have supported me throughout the writing of this book. This project would not have been possible without their guidance, collaboration, and encouragement.

First, I sincerely appreciate my mentors who have guided me at various stages of my career: John Martin, Laura Gunn, and German Molina. Your guidance and collaboration in academic writing and statistical methods helped shape much of the work in this book and have left an indelible mark that will stay with me throughout the remainder of my career (although any errors in this book are certainly my own).

A special thanks to my friend and long-time co-conspirator, Matt Nethery, not only for reading this book cover-to-cover and providing valuable feedback but also for his constant encouragement and camaraderie over the years. From developing iPhone apps in our "younger" years to writing academic papers today, your excitement about learning is infectious. Until the next project!

I also thank my editors, David Grubbs at CRC and Michelle Smith and Shira Evans at O'Reilly, for trusting me to see this work to completion and for their expert guidance that helped shape this work.

I am grateful to the current and past members of the Data Science Team, who influenced me in many ways throughout my career: Sydney Westfall, Drew Tatum, Aiden Choi, Michael Duan, Michael Herron, Tim Lowe, Michael Long, Rachel Turner, Katie Baker, Jacob Horowitz, Donny Shuler, and Taylor Steinberg. I've learned from each and every one of you while working in the trenches together, and your influence is reflected in some capacity in these chapters.

To my professors and peers in DrPH Cohort 4 at The Medical College of Wisconsin, I am beyond grateful to be part of this amazing team and look forward to many more years of learning and growing together. Special thanks to professors David Nelson, Tarakee Jackson, Christopher Simenz, and my incredible cohort: Tiffany Kuo, Daniel Borck, Heidi Moore, Shakari Lewis, Noel Estrada-Merly, Crystal Landeros, Pavneet Banga, Eric Lambert, Lamisa Ashraf, and Andrew Braun. I have never been part of such a supportive and encouraging team. See you all at the finish line in 2027.

I am grateful for the professors and collaborators at UNC-Charlotte— Josh Hertel, Franck Diaz-Garelli, Carly Mahedy, John Reeves, and the late Jeff Meyer and Daniel White—as well as at Penn State Eberly College of Science—Jessica Trail, Allison Deal, and Armine Bagyan. Your contributions have been invaluable to my professional growth.

To my peers and leadership at Premier (past and present) who have influenced or supported me in various capacities, whether through teaching me about healthcare data, policy, coding, or statistics, I thank you (in no particular order): Terri Sawyer, Andy Weber, Parul Vernekar, Chris Stewart, Kelly Larson, Ashley Finke, Ray Perigard, Ben Davis, Ibrokhim Sadikov, Allison Lloyd, Bernie Traiteur, Anna Cheng, Tim Stroupe, Michael Dickson, Ning Rosenthal, Zhun Cao, Marla Kugel, Danielle Lloyd, Eddie Escobar, Alfred Kosgey, Mary Ann Wayer, Travis Cherry, Melissa Medeiros, Louise Zrull, Tedy Rusli, Mike Byndas, Kellie Webb, Steve Cornett, Andrew McAlister, Tasha Lackey, Todd Wilkes, Angela Lanning, Madeleine Biondolillo, Daniel DeBehnke, Apurv Gupta, Lori Harrington, Dena Richardson, Susanne Smiley, Jill Solovey, John Pitsikoulis, Kathy Belk, Kateryna Zakharenko, and Tara Bain.

To my friend Michael Reddington, thank you for sharing your stories and writing process and for motivating me to embark on this journey.

A special thank you goes to Ben Corpuz and the BC Brazilian Jiu-Jitsu team and the staff at Waxhaw Yoga for helping me maintain some semblance of mental stability and balance throughout my career.

I want to express my gratitude to the organizations that support and develop the programming languages and tools essential for modern data analysis. I appreciate the R Foundation for Statistical Computing and The Python Software Foundation for their dedication to advancing R and Python, respectively. I also thank Posit (formerly RStudio) for providing an excellent ecosystem of tools that has made working with R and Python more effective and enjoyable.

To all those mentioned and those who have supported me in any way, I am forever grateful.

1

An Overview of Healthcare Data

Background

When conducting healthcare analyses, we often start with a particular research question or business problem. Perhaps we're interested if patients diagnosed with depression have a decreased risk of readmissions when administered certain antidepressants compared to those undergoing counseling. To conduct this analysis from a tactical perspective, we would need standardized identifiers for medications (antidepressants), diagnoses (depression), services (counseling), and for patients themselves (to identify readmissions) so that the data is consistent across providers. How such concepts are classified can vary considerably depending on the data sources used in our analyses.

Healthcare data is notoriously fragmented and siloed. Each data source has distinct advantages and drawbacks, and the ideal dataset containing a complete narrative of a patient's entire healthcare journey across care settings and payers remains challenging.

In this chapter, we'll discuss the primary data sources available for healthcare analysis. Staying true to the book's scope, as defined in the preface, we'll focus on data centered around the patient—emphasizing data sources that store patient clinical and demographic information and the resulting care provided to them by the healthcare professional. In my experience, the most effective researchers, analysts, statisticians, and data scientists have an intimate understanding of their domain and pesky nuances specific to their datasets. So much of the modeling exercise involves accurate collection and preparation of variables in a way that is most appropriate for the employed statistical model. In my opinion, domain expertise and a firm grasp of the data are just as important as having strong statistical chops.

We can classify patient data into two major groups: EHRs and administrative records. Both data sources capture a wide range of information about the patient encounter, including demographic information, diagnoses, procedures, medications, lab tests, imaging, and services. While there is considerable overlap in information between the two data sources, each is unique and has advantages and disadvantages. A quick reference outlining the data sources discussed here can be found in (Table 1.1).

TABLE 1.1

Common Healthcare Standards for Storing Clinical and Administrative Data

			Administrative			EHR
Standard	Description	Maintainer	UB-04 Inpatient	UB-04 Outpatient	1500	HL7-CDA
ICD-10-CM	Diagnoses	Centers for Disease Control and Prevention's (CDC) National Center for Health Statistics (NCHS).	x	x	x	
ICD-10-PCS	Procedures	Centers for Medicare and Medicaid Services (CMS)	x			
UB-Revenue Codes	Billable items	National Uniform Billing Committee (NUBC)	x	x		
CPT-4	Procedures and other physician services	American Medical Association (AMA)		x	x	
HCPCS	Extends CPT-4 with non-physician services, medications, equipment, and supplies	Centers for Medicare and Medicaid Services (CMS)		x	x	
NDC	Drug products by manufacturer	U.S. Food and Drug Administration (FDA)	x	x	x	

(Continued)

TABLE 1.1 (CONTINUED)

Standard	Description	Maintainer	Administrative			EHR
			UB-04 Inpatient	UB-04 Outpatient	1500	HL7-CDA
SNOMED-CT	Defines hierarchy and relationships across a wide range of clinical concepts (including diagnoses)	SNOMED International				x
LOINC	Defines laboratory and other clinical observations	The Regenstrief Institute with support by the U.S. National Library of Medicine (NLM)				x
RXNORM	Medications and drugs	The National Library of Medicine (NLM)				x

Administrative Data

Hospital administrative data includes a wide range of standardized information about the patient encounter, including transitions to and from the setting of care, demographic information (age, sex, etc.), patient diagnoses and procedures, and billed services and items. Administrative data is collected primarily for billing purposes and can be used to submit claims to payers for reimbursement. Each payer (e.g., Medicare, Medicaid, Cigna, Aeta) has their own requirements specific to the care setting. Medicare, for example, requires hospitalizations to be submitted using a Uniform Billing 04 (UB-04) form and physician offices to be submitted through a 1500 claim form. Data will be extracted from administrative databases to generate a claim in the format required by the payer.

The UB-04 claim form (also known as the 1450 form) stores information about care provided within hospitals and other institutional facilities (e.g., skilled nursing and rehab facilities). Although it is a paper form, most hospitals transmit claims using the electronic 837I (I = Institutional) format. Bear with me, as I know we are approaching terminology overload.

The CMS 1500 claim form, on the other hand, records information about services rendered in a physician's office or outpatient clinic. Like the UB-04 form, it contains patient demographic and clinical information, including diagnoses, services, and procedures. The 1500 form is also paper; however, many physician offices use the 837P (Professional) format to transmit claims electronically.

Given the scope of this book, I will note that a comprehensive review of the hospital billing process and the varying data elements across data sources is not possible. Volumes of technical manuals are available online for those with a much higher pain threshold than me. We will cover what I feel are key data elements often used within healthcare analyses as they relate to the quality and efficiency of patient care. That said, let's discuss the primary data standards typically used to codify clinical information within administrative data across the UB-04 and 1500 forms.

Diagnoses

From a data perspective, a patient has one primary reason for seeking care, captured as a primary or principal diagnosis and, as such, only one principal diagnosis can be recorded on the patient claim. Along with the principal diagnosis, a patient can have multiple secondary diagnoses—peripheral conditions related to the patient's encounter. Secondary diagnoses are further qualified with a present-on-admission (POA) code, indicating if the condition was present on admission or if occurring while in the hospital. The POA status is mainly used in the inpatient setting and is especially helpful when attempting to distinguish preexisting comorbidities from complications that might have resulted from patient care.

Diagnoses are recorded using the International Classification of Diseases (ICD) codes, a coding system integral to healthcare statistics. This discussion will focus on ICD version 10 (ICD-10) codes implemented in the United States in October 2015. Compared to its predecessor, the ICD-9, the ICD-10 system is much more robust and has greater breadth and depth.

The ICD-10 Clinical Modification (ICD-10-CM) family of codes specifically defines patient *diagnoses*. These codes are rich in detail, allowing for a comprehensive representation of a patient's condition. ICD-10-CM codes can range from 3 to 7 characters in length, with the first three positions of the code denoting the broader disease category. The subsequent four positions provide additional information that further qualifies the diagnosis, including details about the disease's site, severity, and etiology (cause). Diagnosis codes can be spliced and truncated to define a group or cross-section of diagnoses across codes.

Category				Etiology, site, and severity			Extension
S	8	3	.	5	1	1	A
The range S80-S89 identifies injuries to the knee and lower leg. Specifically, S83 denotes a dislocation and sprain of joints and ligaments of knee.				S83.5 Sprain of **cruciate** ligament of knee S83.51 Sprain of **anterior cruciate** ligament of knee S83.511 Sprain of **anterior cruciate** ligament of **right** knee			Indicates an initial encounter

FIGURE 1.1
ICD-10 positional components for S83.511A, indicating a sprain of the right knee's anterior cruciate ligament.

For example, consider ICD-10 code S83.511A, which denotes a sprain of the right knee's anterior cruciate ligament. This code goes beyond just identifying a sprain by specifying the location (right knee) and specific ligament (anterior cruciate) related to the injury; it further stipulates that this injury is the first encounter (first occurrence). This level of detail is important for healthcare statisticians and researchers to define narrow cohorts for specific research questions. For example, ICD-10 codes classifying injuries related to the knee and lower leg will be prefixed with codes ranging from S80 to S89. We can drill down further to evaluate only sprains of the cruciate ligament of the knee by evaluating S83 codes. Figure 1.1 shows the levels of specificity for ICD-10-CM code S83.511A, with each digit further qualifying the diagnosis with additional details.

The CMS official guidelines for coding and reporting contain all the gory details (and there are a lot of details) about ICD coding, a punishment reserved only for the highest order of healthcare nerds.

Procedures and Other Services

In a hospital setting, the ICD-10 Procedure Coding System (ICD-10-PCS) is used to classify medical procedures and services, specifically for UB-04 claims. Despite sharing a similar name with ICD-10-CM codes for diseases, ICD-10-PCS serves a different purpose and has its own unique structure.

As shown in Figure 1.2, ICD-10-PCS codes consist of seven alphanumeric characters, each representing a distinct aspect of the procedure. For example, the first character categorizes procedures into broad groups, while the second character specifies the anatomical system or body part involved in the procedure, facilitating research on procedures related to specific anatomical systems. Perhaps the physician used ICD-10-PCS code 0SQC4ZZ to indicate a repair of the right knee joint using an endoscopic approach. We can see in

Section	Body System	Operation	Body Part	Approach	Device	Qualifier
0	S	Q	C	4	Z	Z
Medical and Surgical	Lower Joints	Repair	Right Knee Joint	Percutaneous Endoscopic	No Device	No Qualifier

FIGURE 1.2
Positional components for ICD-10-PCS code 0SQC4ZZ, indicating the repair of a right knee joint using the percutaneous endoscopic approach.

Figure 1.2 the role of each character in the procedure code in adding degrees of specificity related to the procedure.

A related coding system is Current Procedural Terminology Version 4 (CPT-4), not ICD-10-PCS, which defines a comprehensive range of healthcare services and procedures for private and public payers in the outpatient and physician office settings.

CPT-4 codes are represented by a five-digit code ranging from 00100 to 99499 and are categorized based on the type of procedure or service and the relevant anatomical area. Perhaps a patient has a wart removed from their left pinky finger (definitely not talking about myself here), a procedure that would likely be coded with CPT code 17110. This code falls within the broader set of codes related to surgery of the integumentary system. There are two other CPT categories (category II and category III). Category II codes are alphanumeric codes used for performance measurement. These codes are often optional and are not necessary for accurate coding. Category III codes are temporary alphanumeric codes for emerging technology, procedures, and services. The lion's share of coding will occur within the first category of CPT.

CPTs are assigned relative value units (RVUs), which are used to determine payment as part of the MPFS and other private payer models to reimburse physicians for professional services such as those conducted in the physician office setting.

Non-Physician Services

The Healthcare Common Procedure Coding System (HCPCS) was developed by CMS to capture a broader range of services extending beyond the physician services coded in the CPT-4 standard. As such, there are two levels to HCPCS. The first, HCPCS Level I, is simply the CPT-4 coding system, while the second, HCPCS Level II, includes additional codes for non-physician services, medications, equipment, and supplies.

For example, ambulance and other transport services are captured in the A0021 to A0999 range of HCPCS II codes. Within that range, code A0998 indicates an ambulance response and treatment but without transporting the patient.

Revenue Codes

Revenue codes are standardized four-digit numeric codes used in UB-04 data to categorize various services, procedures, and supplies provided by health-care facilities. These codes are primarily used for billing and reimbursement, as they help healthcare payers, such as Medicare, Medicaid, and private insurance companies, understand the types of services and items rendered to patients to determine accurate payment allocation.

Revenue codes convey information such as service categories, locations, levels of care, pharmacy items, laboratory tests, therapeutic treatments, supplies, blood products, psychiatric care, home health services, hospice care, durable medical equipment, rehabilitation, emergency care, and miscellaneous items. Revenue code 0361, for example, indicates that an operating room is utilized for minor surgery.

Drugs and Medications

National Drug Codes (NDCs) are unique identifiers for drugs and medications in the United States and are maintained by the Food and Drug Administration. NDC codes are typically 11 digits in length and are comprised of three components—a four-digit *labeler code* indicating the drug manufacturer, a five-digit *product code* indicating the strength, dose, and drug formulation, and finally, an optional two-digit *package code* indicating the package type and size. This is often referred to as a 5-4-2 structure (labeler code, product code, and package code). Let's look at the NDC 5-4-2 code structure for citalopram, a drug widely used to treat depression. There are several citalopram manufacturers, each with its own NDC labeler code. The two-digit package code is often excluded if we are just interested in the labeler/product code combination. For example, the drug code for citalopram, under the labeler of Allergan, is 0456-4010. This is a manufacturer-specific code for citalopram, marketed as Celexa by Allergan. If we append the two-digit package suffix, we would be referring specifically to a bottle of 100 Celexa film-coated tablets. As shown in Figure 1.3, each part of the NDC code further qualifies the product.

While the NDC code serves as a standardized way to identify drugs and medications uniquely, it is a code specific to the product and not centered around the particular nature of the drug. To identify a drug (opioids, for

Labeler Code (5 digits)	Product Code (4 digits)	Package Code (2 digits)
0456	4010	01
Allergan, Inc.	Celexa (the marketing name for citalopram)	100 film-coated 10 mg tablet in one bottle

FIGURE 1.3
Positional components for NDC code 0456-4010-01, indicating a bottle of 100 Celexa film-coated tablets manufactured by Allergan, Inc.

example) across manufacturers, the researcher would need to identify the list of NDCs across manufacturers to capture all administered opioids. We'll see in the next section that mappings (or crosswalks) exist to facilitate this type of analysis.

Electronic Health Records

As found in the UB-04 and 1500 forms, administrative data is highly standardized for billing and administrative purposes. However, it is mainly limited to data needed for billing and quality improvement. As a result, clinical information unrelated to the billing process will not be recorded in administrative data. The EHR is the upstream source system used by clinical coders to codify diagnoses, procedures, and other patient information for administrative databases. This system contains the granular clinical details of a patient encounter.

EHR data is transactional in nature, reflecting the dynamic nature of patient care. Each interaction with a healthcare provider generates new data entries, resulting in a continuous stream of information. This transactional nature is well-suited for clinical decision-making and real-time patient care but requires aggregation and structuring when conducting patient-level analyses or extracting information over extended periods.

The EHR is notably less standardized than administrative data but is a much richer data source. To address challenges related to interoperability and standardization across EHR systems, healthcare institutions employ Health Level Seven Clinical Document Architecture (HL7 CDA) standards for data exchange. HL7 CDA is a flexible XML (Extensible Markup Language) specification that serves as a bridge between health databases by providing a uniform format for the exchange of clinical documents. While HL7 facilitates interoperability, variations in EHR implementations and local configurations can still introduce challenges in achieving proper data standardization.

The HL7 CDA messaging structure uses several industry standards to capture clinical information such as diagnoses, procedures, orders, results, and medications. Thus, it provides a standard specification and data structure for transmitting established coding systems and hierarchies. In the following sections, we'll focus on some of the more salient coding systems used within the HL7 CDA format.

We've been using the term "standards" loosely in this chapter, but it will be necessary to clarify some terminology before proceeding to the next section. Specifically, we should define two key terms—ontologies and taxonomies.

In healthcare, ontologies are formal, structured representations of complex domain knowledge that define the semantic relationships among medical concepts. The domain knowledge is inherent in the structure of the ontology. For instance, an ontology not only describes the concept of "cardiovascular disease" but may also define its disease subtypes, related risk factors, and the intricate connections between them.

Taxonomies, on the other hand, are hierarchical classification systems used to categorize medical terms, diseases, or procedures at different levels of aggregation. An example of a healthcare taxonomy is the International Classification of Diseases (ICD), which categorizes and codes various diseases and medical conditions for consistent record-keeping and billing purposes.

Regarding the standards discussed in this book, ICD-10-CM, ICD-10-PCS, UB-Revenue Codes, CPT-4, HCPCS, NDC, LOINC, and RXNORM are taxonomies used for categorizing and coding various aspects of healthcare, while SNOMED-CT is an ontology that represents clinical concepts and their semantic relationships in a more comprehensive manner.

SNOMED CT

The Systematized Nomenclature of Medicine—Clinical Terms (SNOMED CT) is an ontology that provides a formal representation of clinical knowledge by defining concepts and relationships within the medical domain. It further includes a hierarchy of clinical concepts and specifies how they relate, making it an incredibly flexible and valuable tool for healthcare systems to represent and share medical knowledge. SNOMED CT is massive as it includes a comprehensive and highly detailed clinical terminology system and provides a standardized way to describe the relationship between clinical information, including diseases, findings, procedures, and more.

If we examine the clinical concept of diabetes mellitus in the SNOMED ontology, we can see that the disease is part of a larger disease hierarchy.

Disorder of body site → disorder of body system → disorder of endocrine system → diabetes mellitus

Note that within SNOMED-CT, a disease might fall within multiple disease hierarchies. Just as diabetes mellitus has multiple "parents" in the hierarchy, it can have multiple "children" in the hierarchy as well (e.g., Types I and II).

Within SNOMED, we not only have an understanding of the various classification levels for the disease, but we also have access to rich information about the relationship between the concept and other clinical concepts. For example, SNOMED-CT provides information regarding associated conditions, underlying conditions, the finding site (part of the body), risk factors, and disease synonyms.

LOINC

Logical Observation Identifiers Names and Codes (LOINC) is a coding system primarily used for laboratory and clinical observations. It standardizes the names and codes for a wide range of laboratory tests, measurements, and clinical observations. Within HL7 CDA, LOINC codes are commonly used to represent laboratory results and observations. A LOINC code, for example, can specify a particular blood test or a clinical measurement like blood pressure.

These codes often capture a question/answer relationship for a medical concept. A physician might order a COVID-19 test for a patient. The LOINC code would be responsible for defining the question, "Does this patient have COVID-19?" in the form of LOINC code 94558-4. As shown in Figure 1.4,

Component (what is being measured?)	Property Characteristics of substance being measured	Time The time interval for the measurement	System The origin of the specimen	Scale Scale indicating quantitative, ordinal, nominal, or narrative	Method The method of measurement employed
SARS coronavirus 2 Ag	PrThr (ordered categorical scale)	Pt (A point-in-time measurement)	Respiratory System Specimen	Ord (Ordinal: Positive/Negative)	IA.rapid (Rapid immunoassay method

FIGURE 1.4
LOINC Code 94558-4 indicating a COVID-19 test.

a LOINC code is uniquely defined by six parts: component, property, time, system, scale, and method.

LOINC 94558-4 tells us that we are conducting a SARS coronavirus two antigen test (component) and that the unit of measurement is an ordered categorical scale (property) from a point-in-time measurement (time). We also know that the test concerns the respiratory system (system), and its result will be expressed on an ordinal scale (scale) using the rapid immunoassay method (method).

While LOINC code 94558-4 is a question (does this patient have COVID-19?), the answer is represented by another LOINC list code, LL2021-5, which defines a list of positive, negative, or invalid answers. Note that while the list of possible answers is defined as LL2021-5, the answer values for positive, negative, and invalid are also assigned their own LOINC code of LA6576-8, LA6577-6, and LA15841-2, respectively.

RxNorm

RxNorm is a standardized terminology system specifically designed to identify medications and drugs and used within the HL7 CDA specification. It provides codes and names for clinical drugs, including generic and brand names, strengths, and forms. Unlike NDC codes, RxNorm codes include information about drug classes and relationships between different drug entities.

Drugs and medications within RxNorm are identified by an Rx Concept Unique Identifier (RxCUI) code, made unique through the combination of the active ingredient, strength, and dosage form. These components can be seen in the RxCUI standardized description and will take the form <drug><strength/dose><dosage form>. RxNorm also contains one-to-many mappings from an RxCUI to NDC code, allowing the user a homogenous definition of a drug across NDC codes.

In the section on NDC codes, we defined Celexa (generic citalopram) 10 mg tablet as NDC 0456-4010-01. An equivalent code of the RxNorm system is RxCUI code 284591. Within the RxNorm system, we not only identify this drug as a citalopram 10 mg tablet, but we also know that the active ingredient is citalopram, which is part of the drug class of selective serotonin reuptake inhibitors (SSRIs). The description of the RxCUI 284591 is citalopram 10 mg oral tablet, in compliance with the standardized format (Figure 1.5).

Drug	Strength/Dose	Dosage Form
Citalopram	10 mg	Oral Tablet

FIGURE 1.5
RxCUI code 284591 indicating a Citalopram 10 mg oral tablet.

RxNorm is centered around the drug rather than the product (as with NDC codes). As such, it helps identify drugs based on their active ingredient across manufacturers and dosage forms. It further allows the researcher to understand how drugs relate to the broader classification.

Other Healthcare Data Sources

While we've touched on some common sources and data formats used to capture patient-centered data, it will be helpful to touch on some tangential data sources that are important for healthcare analyses.

Hospital Information

When conducting healthcare analyses, we are often interested in structural information about the hospital where care was provided. For example, we might be interested in whether a teaching or academic hospital generally provides higher-quality care for COPD patients than non-teaching or academic facilities. The number of beds, its location, whether urban or rural, or access to equipment could better inform our patient-level analysis.

Various organizations provide hospital information, but we'll discuss two of the most notable here.

Centers for Medicare and Medicaid Services (CMS)

Any hospital that accepts Medicare insurance (nearly all hospitals) will be assigned a CMS certification number (CCN). The CCN is a six-digit number with the first two digits representing the U.S. state or territory and the last four digits representing the type of facility (e.g., psychiatric, rehab, skilled nursing facility, short-term hospital). CMS provides a wide range of datasets related to quality and payment. A few worth noting are the CMS cost report, the CMS IPPS Impact file, and the CMS Care Compare database.

The CMS Cost Report is a financial document submitted by healthcare providers participating in the Medicare and Medicaid programs. While these reports are an essential part of the CMS reimbursement process, they are also an excellent source for obtaining hospital-level information, including the location, types of beds and their respective bed counts, number of discharges, income, and total staff salary cost (https://data.cms.gov/provider-compliance/cost-report/hospital-provider-cost-report/data).

The CMS Impact file drives Medicare payment and includes rich information about a hospital, including ownership status, case mix, region, hospital type, beds, and census (https://www.cms.gov/medicare/payment/prospective-payment-systems/acute-inpatient-pps/fy-2024-ipps-final-rule-home-page).

The Care Compare data catalog includes rich databases across many care settings. Here, one can find a wide range of quality and efficiency measures for hospitals, physician offices, and other care settings. In many of these databases, CMS consolidates data from disparate agencies so that information about an organization's performance is centrally located.

American Hospital Association (AHA)

The AHA surveys hospitals and other healthcare organizations with detailed questionnaires, collecting data on hospital operations, finances, staffing, services offered, and more. The AHA survey captures beyond what can be found in the CMS data sources. For example, through the AHA data, we identify hospitals that have a fertility clinic, conduct robotic surgery, or provide chemotherapy treatment (https://www.ahadata.com/system/files/media/file/2023/09/AHA-Annual-Survey.pdf).

Physicians and Organizations

The National Provider ID (NPI) from the CMS *National Plan and Provider Enumeration System (NPPES)* is perhaps the most well-known identifier for physicians and organizations. NPI codes are ten-digit codes grouped into individuals (I) or organizations (O), each with information specific to that entity type. NPIs can uniquely identify individuals and organizations across payers and care settings and are helpful in understanding a patient's interaction with a care provider throughout their care episode.

The NPI data includes high-level information about the provider and up to 15 standardized specialties (which the NPPES refers to as taxonomies). Of the 15 possible specialties, only one is identified as a primary specialty. NPI codes can be found within administrative data and EHR systems and are the most universal identifier for care providers.

Social and Environmental Data

Often, the data available within the patient databases (EHR or administrative) do not capture the breadth of data needed for our analysis. There are cases where we are interested in more information about the patient's social and environmental circumstances of the patient. In these cases, we must seek outside datasets to extend the patient-centered data.

Given that this topic is moving beyond healthcare to a broader dataset about specific geographic regions, there will be countless data sources that may be useful, and their relevancy will depend on the particular research question. We might be interested in crime statistics, environmental issues (such as air and water quality), socioeconomic status data (such as income and home value), or economic data (cost of living, wage indices, etc.).

Of the many datasets we could discuss, those related to social drivers (or determinants) of health SDoH are perhaps the most salient. SDoH refers to the social, economic, and environmental factors that influence a person's overall health and well-being. These determinants can significantly impact an individual's healthcare access, risk of developing certain health conditions, and overall quality of life. A few of the most notable data sources include the CDC Agency for Toxic Substances and Disease Registry Social Vulnerability dataset, the AHRQ SDoH dataset, the Area Deprivation Index (ADI), and the Minority Health Social Vulnerability dataset from the Health and Human Services Office of Minority Health. A broader, more expansive dataset is the Area Health Resource File, which contains consolidated information sourced across many organizations and domains. Studies have shown that variation in quality is often partially explained by circumstances outside of the hospital, so adjusting for factors related to a patient's environment can often help produce more accurate statistical analyses. Resources for these datasets can be found at the end of this chapter.

While we discussed some of the most used data sources in healthcare research, it is far from a comprehensive list. Hospitals and third-party organizations collect patient survey data on their health, lifestyle, or satisfaction with their care provider. There are disease registries—specialized databases designed to track specific diseases, such as cancer or diabetes, and to monitor prevalence and outcomes. Vital statistics databases contain birth and death certificates, demographic information, and cause-of-death information. Remote health monitoring devices and telehealth visits store real-time health information.

Public Use Datasets

Various research databases containing administrative or EHR data are available online, for free or for a fee. Rather than listing the many data sources here, I'll direct readers to a resource from John Hopkin's Welch

Medical Library that catalogs several useful databases. Of special note are the HCUP National Inpatient Sample (NIS) and MedPAR databases, which are rich sources of administrative data regularly used in research and publications.

Additional Resources

AHRQ SDoH Database. https://www.ahrq.gov/sdoh/index.html

Area Deprivation Index. https://www.neighborhoodatlas.medicine.wisc.edu/

CDC/ATSDR Social Vulnerability Index. https://www.atsdr.cdc.gov/placeand health/svi/index.html

HCUP Databases. https://hcup-us.ahrq.gov/databases.jsp

HHS Area Health Resource File. https://data.hrsa.gov/topics/health-workforce/ ahrf

MEDPAR. https://www.cms.gov/data-research/files-for-order/limited-data-set-lds-files

Minority Health SVI. https://www.minorityhealth.hhs.gov/minority-health-svi/

2

Healthcare Measures

Measurement in healthcare is deceivingly complicated. Let's consider the great diversity of human illness (both mental and physical), the range of care settings in which a patient can receive care, and the numerous stakeholders (patients, physicians, hospitals, regulatory agencies, and payers). It should not be surprising that there are, quite literally, thousands of healthcare measures designed to measure various aspects of care. In this chapter, we'll discuss key components of measure development, followed by a discussion of standard industry measures and measure sets used in healthcare statistics.

Measure development is critical to healthcare statistics, as statisticians and data scientists are often tasked with developing measures specific to a targeted research area. This process can be challenging, and there are many pitfalls. To create a measure, we must first determine what we are measuring. Typically, healthcare measures are grouped into five main categories: outcomes, process, patient experience, efficiency, and structural.

Types of Measures

Let's take a closer look at each of these categories.

Outcome Measures

Outcome measures are perhaps the most prolific measures in healthcare, as they capture the potential adverse results of patient care. This group includes measures such as mortality, readmissions, and complications.

DOI: 10.1201/9781003609759-2

Additional measures such as patient cost or length of stay are often referred to as outcome measures but are primarily designed to measure the efficiency of care. Outcome measures are also some of the most challenging to develop, as the expectation of an outcome will vary based on the patient's unique clinical and demographic characteristics. We would certainly expect an 87-year-old man with severe osteoarthritis and type II diabetes, for example, to be more prone to pressure ulcers (bed sores) than a 23-year-old male with no chronic conditions. Therefore, in developing outcome measures, it is important to "risk adjust" or "risk standardize" the measures to account for patient characteristics that might affect our expectation of an outcome. We discussed this topic in greater detail in the chapter on standardization; however, for now, recall that most risk-adjusted measures are designed to compare some observed event (e.g., a complication) to an expectation of the event based on the patient's characteristics. When evaluating the outcomes for a patient population, the total number of observed events (e.g., total pressure ulcers) is compared to the total number of expected events (e.g., the total number of pressure ulcers that we would expect from the evaluated population) in the form of a ratio. This ratio is typically abbreviated as an O/E. O/E ratios greater than 1 indicate more cases than expected, given the evaluated patients, while O/E ratios less than 1 indicate fewer cases than expected. Risk standardized measures such as those expressed as an O/E ratio are designed to fairly compare performance across physicians, facilities, and other levels of data so that they are not unfairly penalized for having adverse events beyond those expected, given the unique nature of the patient population.

Mortality

Mortality, or death, is perhaps the most prominent measure in healthcare analysis, as it is the ultimate outcome that patient care is designed to prevent. Incidence of mortality can be measured as inpatient mortality or episodic mortality. In the former case, mortality is identified if it occurs during the inpatient stay. This is a direct measure and more immediate measure of mortality, and given that the event is recorded within the scope of the encounter, it is typically a more reliable measure. For example, within administrative data, we can identify mortality through a standardized discharge status, and within the EHR, it is recorded through the date of death. A drawback of the inpatient mortality measure is that it does not capture potential deaths that occur after the patient is discharged. Hospitals that prematurely discharge patients without the most complete care might have higher rates of mortality within an episode but lower mortality within the inpatient setting. Therefore, mortality is often measured as 30-day mortality (sometimes longer), using additional data (such as Medicare enrollment data or vital statistics) to identify death outside of the hospital. While 30-day mortality is a more complete measure from a care perspective, it can be challenging to calculate from a data integration perspective.

Standard industry mortality measures are the Yale Center for Outcomes Research & Evaluation (CORE) 30-day risk-standardized mortality measure and the AHRQ inpatient mortality measure set, which includes Inpatient Quality Indicators (IQIs) specific to certain medical and procedure groups.

Readmissions

Readmission measures refer to patients returning to the hospital after discharge—a sign of potentially incomplete care from the previous stay. With readmissions, an "index visit" is identified, which marks the beginning of an episode. Typically, readmissions are measured within 30 days (like mortality) but can be evaluated within 60 or 90 days, depending on the research question. There are many nuances to a robust readmissions measure. For example, processing steps might be taken to ensure that only one readmission is counted if a patient is admitted multiple times within the evaluated episode (e.g., 30 days).

Additionally, a distinction between planned and unplanned readmissions might be made within the measure definition. Arguably, a COVID-19 patient discharged from an ICU but returning two weeks later with a broken hip is not an indicator of suboptimal care (unless there was an adverse drug event from the previous stay, for example). Entire industry algorithms exist to distinguish planned and unplanned readmission.

As with 30-day mortality, calculating readmissions can be challenging from a data perspective. Hospitals attempting to calculate readmissions using their own data will be blind to readmissions occurring outside the hospital. A patient discharged from one facility (or system) may be readmitted to a hospital in the same region. Depending on hospital market share, readmission rates can vary (regardless of quality). A small rural hospital might be the only hospital in their area and will receive almost all readmissions to their hospital.

In contrast, an urban hospital in a population-dense region might experience a greater proportion of readmissions outside the scope of its data. Such issues with data linkage are discussed later in this chapter in the section on patient identifiers. Yale CORE also calculates 30-day risk-standardized readmission measures used within various publicly regulated programs.

Complications

Complications might be the most complex measure to evaluate. They can be calculated within administrative data or through the EHR, and industry-standard measures have been developed for both data sources. For example, the National Healthcare Safety Network (NHSN) calculates various health-care-associated infections (HAIs) using data sourced directly from the EHR, which CMS publicly reports. Examples of these measures include incidences of Methicillin-resistant Staphylococcus aureus (MRSA), Clostridioides difficile (C. diff), infections related to central lines and catheters, and surgical site infections. Industry complication measure sets using administrative data include the AHRQ Patient Safety Indicators, CMS Hospital Acquired Conditions, and the Yale CORE episodic complication measures.

Complications are incredibly diverse and are often grouped into medical and surgical categories. Surgical complications might include accidental cuts and lacerations during surgery or a surgical instrument left within the patient after surgery. Examples of medical complications include various types of wound infections, adverse drug events, and accidental falls. Complications represent many facets of care and require nuanced inclusion and exclusion criteria. We should not reward physicians for having zero accidental punctures, for example, when they do not conduct surgeries.

Similarly, a hospital ward that does not use central lines should not be rewarded for having zero central line-associated bloodstream infections (CLABSIs). Furthermore, a physician should not be penalized for a catheter-associated urinary tract infection (CAUTI) identified on the first day of a patient's stay, as the bacterial infection could not have been cultured in one day (indicating that it was present on admission). When constructing individual complication measures, it is important to identify clinically relevant patients and the conditions specific to the complication being evaluated.

Process Measures

Process measures are designed to measure consistency with evidence-based practices. One of the most well-known process measures evaluates aspirin administration on arrival for AMI patients. This measure is part of a set of "core measures" defined by the Joint Commission. While outcome measures are typically risk-adjusted—given the varying expectations of an outcome based on patient characteristics—process measures are typically measured as a binary occurrence: that is, a process was either followed or not, regardless of patient characteristics.

Process measures are usually expressed as a numerator over a denominator, where the denominator defines the specific eligibility criteria for the measure. For the aspirin on arrival measure (AMI-1), a patient must satisfy the measure's denominator eligibility criteria with characteristics such as having AMI (based on ICD-10-CM coding), age 18 or older, and not being discharged on the day of arrival. The measure also excludes patients in the event of aspirin contraindication (e.g., a patient is already on a blood thinner, and an additional dose of aspirin could be dangerous). The numerator is the administration of aspirin within 24 hours before or after arrival. Along with the measure, the Joint Commission provides a clinical rationale, further corroborated by various academic sources justifying the approach as evidence-based.

There is a cornucopia of process measures defined through several industry-standard measure sets. Such measures can be more general in nature or specific to a physician's specialty or practice. An ophthalmologist might use a measure on dilated macular examinations for patients 50 years or older with macular degeneration. A dentist might measure the proportion of patients ages 6–20 receiving fluoride varnish during their dental examination, and mental health professionals might be measured by the rate of suicide risk assessments for patients 18 years and older diagnosed with major depressive disorder.

Patient Reported Outcomes

As you might have guessed, patient-reported outcomes are, in fact, outcomes reported by the patient. Such outcomes can include, for example, a patient's self-reported pain levels, functional status (i.e., the ability to perform certain activities), and satisfaction following care. They are used within various regulatory programs (e.g., MIPS, Hospital Value-Based Purchasing [HVBP] program, and the CMS Overall Star Ratings program) and can impact physician and hospital payments from CMS and other payers.

Patient experience measures are perhaps the most well-known patient-reported outcomes. Data for patient experience measures are typically captured through phone calls, paper surveys, or electronic surveys conducted by a third-party organization. Chances are, you've received an email or letter containing a patient satisfaction survey after visiting a physician's office or hospital. The questions are designed to measure various dimensions of a patient's experience during care, such as timeliness of care of appointments, nurse and doctor communication, and cleanliness and quietness of the hospital. Within the physician office setting, the AHRQ Consumer Assessment of Healthcare Providers and Systems (CAHPS) survey is commonly used, while in the inpatient setting, the Hospital Consumer Assessment of Healthcare Providers and Systems (HCAHPS) survey is employed.

Efficiency Measures

Efficiency measures are designed to identify opportunities for process optimization, care coordination, cost containment, and resource efficiency. This section will explore several key efficiency measures used in healthcare data analyses and measurement.

Cost

Cost is often considered an efficiency measure as it refers to the cost of care incurred by the healthcare provider (e.g., a hospital). It is typically a measure designed to balance the resources expended and the outcomes achieved. These measures encompass not only direct costs of care (e.g., supplies, blood, drugs) but also indirect costs such as administrative overhead (e.g., labor, utilities, facilities). Evaluating cost efficiency helps healthcare organizations allocate resources effectively and identify opportunities to change processes or renegotiate the costs of supplies. In many cases, cost is a severity-adjusted (or risk-standardized) measure, as the expectation of cost for a patient during an inpatient stay or larger clinical episode will vary depending on the patient's clinical and demographic characteristics. Therefore, cost can be measured as a ratio of observed cost to expected cost.

Length of Stay

The length of a patient's hospital stay (LOS) is a prominent measure of healthcare efficiency. Shorter hospital stays, without compromising the quality of care, often translate to cost savings and improved patient experiences. Efficiency measures related to LOS evaluate whether patients are hospitalized for an appropriate duration, considering their specific medical conditions and treatment needs. As with cost, LOS is typically risk-standardized to account for the patient mix within an evaluated population.

Utilization

Efficiency measures can also evaluate the reasonable and appropriate usage of resources such as supplies, tests, and medications. The Healthcare Effectiveness Data and Information Set (HEDIS) measure set published by the National Committee for Quality Assurance (NCQA) includes a wide range of measures related to overuse and appropriateness of resources. For example, the "Use of Imaging Studies in Low Back Pain" measure is an evidence-based measure that assesses potential overuse of imaging services (such as X-rays, MRIs, and CT scans) for patients with lower back pain—as unnecessary use of such imaging has not been shown to result in improved patient outcomes and further exposes can expose patient to undue and potentially harmful radiation. Other measures may evaluate excessive or unnecessary use of medications (such as antibiotics or opioids), imaging, labs, and other costly services.

Perhaps the most well-known measure of utilization is the Medicare Spending Per Beneficiary Measure (MSPB), designed to assess risk-adjusted episodic Medicare cost—that is, the amount that Medicare reimburses for the entire patient episode. The MSPB measure episode is initiated with an index visit to a hospital, resulting in an episode window ranging from three days before the index and 30 after discharge. The measure evaluates all Medicare payments for a given patient within that episode and assesses if the total episodic utilization is more than we would expect on average. The intuition behind the measure is that improved care coordination across care settings will result in less overall utilization. The MSPB measure is especially impactful for clinicians and hospitals as it is included in CMS regulatory programs designed to incentivize quality and efficiency through potential reductions in Medicare payments. It is a complex measure with many nuances and is challenging for hospitals and physicians to improve.

Structural Measures

Lastly are structural measures, which are pivotal in evaluating and improving the quality and efficiency of healthcare delivery. Structural measures are typically assessed at the organizational level and include labor-related measures (nurse-to-patient ratios, the percentage of contract labor on a hospital unit, bed occupancy rates) and interoperability (adoption of technology standards, and implementation of EHR-based reporting). While structural measures are ultimately intended to improve the quality and efficiency of care, they are often implemented in pursuit of various accreditation and certifications—such as those provided by the Joint Commission.

In the above paragraphs, we've discussed a wide range of measure sets maintained by various organizations. Table 2.1 lists some of the most commonly employed healthcare measure sets.

Measure Development

As healthcare analysts, we are often tasked with developing measures outside of the selection of industry-standard measures discussed above. In this section, we'll discuss essential aspects of custom measure development.

TABLE 2.1

Common Industry Measure Sets

Measure Steward	Measure Set	Measure Types	Data Source
Yale Center for Outcomes Research and Evaluation (CORE)	Risk Standardized Inpatient Outcomes	Outcomes	Administrative, EHR
Agency for Healthcare Research and Quality (AHRQ)	IQIs and Patient Safety Indicators (PSI)	Outcomes	Administrative
The Joint Commission	Core Measures	Process, Outcome, Structural	Administrative, EHR
Centers for Medicare and Medicaid Services (CMS)	Healthcare Acquired Conditions (HACs)	Outcomes	Administrative
Centers for Medicare and Medicaid Services (CMS)	Medicare Spending Per Beneficiary (MSPB)	Efficiency	Administrative
National Committee for Quality Assurance (NCQA)	Healthcare Effectiveness Data and Information Set (HEDIS)	Process, Efficiency	Administrative
National Healthcare Safety Network (NHSN)	Healthcare-Associated Infections (HAI)	Outcomes	EHR
Hospital Consumer Assessment of Healthcare Providers and Systems (HCAHPS) for hospitals and the	Patient Satisfaction	Patient Reported	Survey
Consumer Assessment of Healthcare Providers and Systems (CAHPS)	Patient Satisfaction	Patient Reported	Survey

Cohort Criteria

Once the measure concept has been determined (e.g., mortality, hemoglobin A1C, patient discharge instructions, pressure ulcers), the inclusion and exclusion criteria for the patient population can be defined. Perhaps we've created a measure that evaluates mothers who have returned to the emergency department within 30 days after delivering a newborn. In the measure definition, we must define the characteristics qualifying a patient for the measure. Perhaps we use the patient's MS-DRG or specific ICD-10 codes to identify delivering mothers. We might also set age ranges to exclude patients outside a normal delivery range.

Often, measures are used to evaluate the performance of clinicians, hospitals, and other care providers, so it is important to think about what is within the control of the care provider. For example, if a patient leaves the hospital AMA (against medical advice), the physician might not have had the opportunity to provide the full extent of care. If such patients were included in the measure, would the physician be unfairly penalized for an unfavorable outcome for that patient? Imagine a hospital administrator discussing with a physician how their AMA patient did not receive adequate discharge instructions as part of their patient experience survey. Similarly, we could consider patients under DNR (do not resuscitate) status. Should DNR patients who expire in the hospital be evaluated equally with those who are not DNR—especially considering that extreme rescue measures will not occur for the DNR patient (compared to the DNR patient)? A patient's transfer-in and transfer-out status should also be considered. Imagine a patient being transferred to a hospital with a CLABSI and who subsequently dies while in the hospital. Should the admitting hospital be penalized for an outcome due to care provided mainly by the transferring facility? While much of the cohort identification process is about identifying patients satisfying the clinical definition of the measure, there is also a fairness component so that care providers are not unfairly penalized for outcomes outside of their control. As we'll see in the chapter on risk adjustment, these considerations do not always need to be handled through exclusion rules, as some of these factors can be handled as confounding variables within the statistical models in the development of risk-adjusted outcomes. We'll discuss this in more detail in the chapter on Standardization (Chapter 8).

Data Standardization

Another challenging aspect of measure development is obtaining a standardized and stable definition for diseases, procedures, and other healthcare concepts. But Mike, can't we use standards like ICD-10 to classify clinical concepts in a consistent manner? Unfortunately, the answer in many cases is no. Coding standards are continually evolving and being refined by stewards of those standards. ICD-10 codes, for example, are now updated twice annually. In that process, ICD-10 codes can be replaced with new ones (e.g., one code might be broken out into three for greater specificity). The same is true for MS-DRG and CPT-4 codes. As such, there is a shelf-life to measure definitions. A measure using a disease definition based on the current ICD-10 standards can produce misleading results if applied to a different timeframe, as the way a disease is defined today through ICD-10 coding may be very different from how it was defined in the past. Therefore, regularly maintaining measure definitions is necessary to ensure that the results remain valid.

One way to mitigate some of the effects of changing standards is to classify diseases more broadly such that the broader definition absorbs granular changes in standards for highly specific codes. Perhaps we are evaluating osteoarthritis as a risk factor for total hip and knee complications. Many ICD-10 codes define various types and locations of arthritis, and these specific codes are subject to change as the ICD-10 coding system is updated. If we were to group all forms of arthritis into a broader category, changes in the specific codes would not affect our more generalized definition (of course, any underlying mappings would need to be maintained to ensure that the new codes are mapped to the broader category).

In this section, we'll focus on administrative coding, one of the most standardized sources for diagnoses and procedures regularly used in healthcare analyses.

Diagnosis and Procedure Classification

Let's talk about some ways that one might choose to categorize diseases and procedures.

We've touched on MS-DRGs in the previous chapter, but discussing their use in healthcare research and statistics will be helpful. It is important to know that MS-DRGs are a grouping defined for reimbursement from Medicare. It is essentially a grouping of related conditions that fall within a similar cost category. Each patient encounter is assigned only one MS-DRG, which is a grouping based primarily on the patient's principal diagnoses. MS-DRGs are classified as medical or surgical types and provide additional information related to other clinical conditions that have occurred with that patient encounter. This said, cost is the primary driver of an MS-DRG grouping. Like ICD-10 codes, MS-DRG codes (and their grouping rules) change at regular intervals and are subject to change over time. MS-DRGs can be further grouped into one of 25 Major Diagnostic Related Categories (MDC) for a broad categorization of MS-DRGs.

Additionally, it is common practice to average the MS-DRGs based on their MS-DRG weight to form a Case Mix Index (CMI). A CMI can be calculated at various levels (e.g., physician, service line, or hospital) and is often used to capture the relative complexity of a patient population. While the MS-DRG is often used as a clinical grouping in health research and statistics, there are alternatives that are better suited for grouping related clinical conditions.

One of the most common standards for grouping clinical conditions is the AHRQ Clinical Classification Software Refined (CCSR) groupings for diagnoses and procedures. Using the CCSR standard, ICD-10-CM codes are grouped into 530 disease categories and 22 body systems, and ICD-10-PCS codes are grouped into 320 procedure categories across 31 clinical domains. CCSR codes can greatly simplify the measure development process by grouping related conditions into comorbidities and complications as part of the larger measure development process.

Another grouping for diagnoses commonly employed in measure development is the Hierarchical Condition Categories (HCC). HCCs were developed by CMS as part of Medicare Advantage (where private insurance companies contract with the federal government to provide Medicare benefits) but are often used to group ICD-10-CM diagnoses into 115 HCCs (at the time of this publication).

For a more robust, flexible mapping, one might consider the Unified Medical Language System (UMLS) meta-thesaurus maintained by the U.S. National Library of Medicine. The UML meta-thesaurus is designed to unify the many healthcare taxonomies and ontologies to find equivalency across various clinical concepts. Within the meta-thesaurus, mappings between SNOMED-CT and ICD-10-CM are available, allowing researchers to define ICD-10 codes across the robust SNOMED-CT ontology. Similarly, ICD-10-PCS and CPT-4 codes can be evaluated within the SNOMED-CT ontology for more dynamic procedure classification. As with all analyses, there are tradeoffs between complexity and efficiency.

Within the broader category of disease classification, industry-standard definitions exist for classifying ICD-10-CM-based comorbidities that may increase a patient's risk for adverse outcomes. Two noteworthy comorbidity standards are the Charlson and Elexhauser comorbidities. The Charlson and Elixhauser comorbidities are often expressed as an index aggregating the collective risk across individual patient comorbidities. AHRQ further publishes a Chronic Condition Indicator Refined (CCIR) list that designates specific diagnoses as chronic conditions.

The literature contains many domain-specific comorbidity definitions, and their utility and relevance will depend on the research question being addressed.

There are tradeoffs in generalized definitions for diseases and procedures. A definition that is too broad will lose important clinical specificity when assessing risk, while a definition that is too narrow may not be useful (due to low volume) and is at greater risk of being influenced by changes in coding standards. Finding the right level of definition is an art; if done well, it can result in a much more reliable measure over time.

Identifying Patients

Uniquely identifying patients allows researchers to track them across the continuum of care, whether to assess the cost of an episode of care across care settings or identify readmissions, mortality, and complications occurring post-discharge.

There are several ways that a patient can be identified within healthcare data, but typically, it will be through one of three codes—a medical record number (MRN), a beneficiary ID, or a master person ID (MPI). There are, like all datasets, tradeoffs with each of these.

The MRN is a unique patient identifier with a given hospital or health system, but it is not unique across health systems and care settings. As a result, it provides incomplete information about a patient's journey. Therefore, using an MRN to calculate readmissions or 30-day mortality will only provide visibility into events that occur within the scope of that data. For example, a patient discharged from Health System A and readmitted to Health System B may not be visible to the analyst using an MRN number (given that the code is specific to Health System A).

Another identifier is the beneficiary ID, which is assigned by the payer (the insurance company). The beneficiary ID will remain the same for a patient across systems and care settings and is a more robust ID for measuring care across the continuum. The drawback, of course, is that a payer represents a cross-section of the patient population. Medicare and Medicaid are two of the largest payers in the United States, and their data is regularly used in analyses, given that they can be purchased under license from CMS. The drawback, however, is that Medicare includes data for patients primarily 65 or older (with some exceptions), and Medicaid represents a cross-section of the population with low income or who are disabled. While linking on beneficiary ID provides a more complete picture of a single patient, it often captures a narrow segment of the larger patient population.

The holy grail of identifiers is the MPI—an identifier assigned to patients that is unique across payers and care settings. MPIs are typically generated using sophisticated matching algorithms that match patients based on their name, address, date of birth, and other identifying characteristics. The MPI process is notoriously difficult and is almost always a probabilistic-based match. While we might be confident that 97-year-old Rufus Beelzebub Wasowski in Lubbock, TX, in one hospital is the same as Rufus Beelzebub Wasowski in Lubbock, TX, seen in another hospital, we might be less confident about John Smith in Manhattan matching another John Smith in Manhattan. The ability to produce a high confidence MPI value often requires detailed patient information often unavailable in research datasets. There is no perfection in MPI identification, and a researcher should know that MPIs typically come with some degree of error.

Clinical Episodes

Related to patient identification is the idea of a clinical episode—a range of time relevant to the condition being evaluated. While many measures evaluate performance using data limited to what is available at the point of care (e.g., inpatient mortality, Hemoglobin 1AC), other measures require evaluating patients longitudinally across care settings. We might consider the total 90 cost of an AMI episode. Using a unique patient identifier (a beneficiary ID, perhaps), we might sum the total cost across physician office, inpatient, and outpatient data to determine episodic cost. When developing measures, it is necessary to consider a timeframe relevant to a given measure. These cross-cutting or continuum-based measures are becoming more common as the eye of healthcare analysis looks beyond the siloed care settings toward the broader overall care provided to a patient.

A representative example of this is mortality. While inpatient mortality is often reported as an immediate measure of quality of care, a patient discharged too soon without receiving adequate care may expire at home or in another care setting. Therefore, it is important to measure both inpatient mortality and mortality within some follow-up period (episode) in which the patient is sensitive to the care provided during their previous stay.

Some researchers and healthcare organizations employ episode groupers that group patient encounters into a broader time grouping or episode. Typically, these algorithms include an index visit (an initial visit that marks the start of the episode), which anchors the episode relative to the care provided before and after the visit.

Attribution

Physician attribution is the process or method by which physicians are attributed to patients as being responsible for a patient's care. Despite being an understudied aspect of healthcare analysis, attribution methods are necessary so that physicians are not unfairly attributed to adverse events or excess utilization for which they had little involvement.

We can group attribution methods into two categories: plurality and inpatient attribution.

Plurality attribution is designed to identify the physician responsible for a patient across care settings within some episode. The episode could be based on a specific diagnosis (a 60-day pneumonia episode, for example) or across a set timeframe. These methods commonly work by identifying the physician associated with the plurality (i.e., the highest count) of visits or the highest total cost within the episode. Perhaps a patient saw the primary care provider (PCP) three times, went to the emergency department (ED) once, and was admitted to a med/surg unit twice within one year. If the total number of visits is used, the PCP would be attributed; however, an inpatient physician could be responsible for the larger episode if the total cost is used. Generally however, the attributed physician in these models is the PCP.

In the inpatient setting, a patient may be seen by multiple physicians with different specialties and varying durations. Consider a patient with an incidence of retained surgical bodies (RSBs) after surgery—a complication where the surgeon inadvertently leaves an object in the patient, such as a sponge, after surgery. Let's also say that this patient developed a CAUTI while recovering in the med/surg ward. This patient was seen by two hospitalists and a surgeon. In an ideal world, the RSB would be attributed to the surgeon as most responsible for this avoidable complication. The CAUTI incident is a bit more complicated. It could be argued that the hospitalist physician should be attributed to the CAUTI incident, but such infections are generally a result of poor hygienic practices and are more sensitive to nursing care. If selecting the hospitalist, we would need to decide if both should be attributed or perhaps we would attribute the physician who saw the patient with the greatest duration of time.

Attribution is, I might say, "complicated", and physicians and hospitals can employ several methods to make more informed attribution assignments. Some methods use fixed business rules, while others use statistical modeling to make a probabilistic assignment.

Coding and Documentation

In any analysis, we should be cautious about how much trust we put into the data. Humans can enter inaccurate or incomplete data into the EHR or neglect to enter important information altogether. Incorrect or missing data can be a source information bias, where the data does not accurately represent reality. One area where we must be especially careful is the standardization of clinical concepts like diagnoses and procedures. Coding ICD-10 codes and HCPCS/CPT4 codes is primarily a human process (although computer-assisted coding tools are becoming more common), making it prone to error.

Beyond the discussion of errors that can occur in the clinical coding process, the concepts of coding intensity and coding specificity should be touched upon. It is important to remember that the clinical coding process is motivated by reimbursement from a payer (such as Medicare) and that clinical information irrelevant to reimbursement (e.g., smoking cessation, aspects of SDoH) might not be recorded in the administrative data. Therefore, there is a point in abstracting patient information where the hospital or physician's office will receive no additional payment for added coding. For example, perhaps a patient is admitted to the hospital with Acute Myocardial Infarction but also has Type II diabetes and a history of prostate cancer. At a certain point, the reimbursement for the claim generated from this data will not increase, even if additional details about the patient are recorded. As a result, there is, quite literally, no payoff for the extra coding work.

Deficits in coding rigor can occur in two ways. First is the concept of coding intensity, where the clinical coder neglects to capture the breadth of information about a patient encounter. The second relates to coding specificity, which results from a clinical coder neglecting to fully qualify the code to the highest degree of specificity possible. Coding specificity is typically measured by the proportion of ICD-10 codes that are "unspecified". In other words, the coder selected a broad catch-all ICD-10 code to represent the condition (e.g., "unspecified dementia"). While coding intensity is related to the quantity (or breadth) of coding, coding intensity relates to the quality (or depth) of coding. Variation in coding intensity and specificity can affect the validity of a measure if corrections are not in place to ensure measure comparability across healthcare organizations.

Balancing Measures

We should not evaluate measures in a vacuum. When developing measures, it is important to consider how improvement in one measure might affect the broader picture of patient care. For example, what is the interaction between a hospital's cost-cutting measure and patient morbidity? Does cost-cutting affect the quality of care? Does increasing nurse-to-patient ratios increase nursing burnout? If patients are discharged from the hospital prematurely, do readmission rates increase?

The point here is that care should be evaluated holistically so that improvement in one measure does not result in an unfavorable result in another. Balancing measures are designed to mitigate the problem (i.e., the overemphasis of one measure over another). One recent extreme example occurred with the HCAHPS patient satisfaction survey, where patients were asked if their pain was adequately controlled. As background, this measure at the time was used within CMS regulatory programs that would financially incentivize hospitals to perform well, and so poor performance on any measure was evaluated with scrutiny. At the time, around 2016, there was increasing awareness of the opioid crisis, and in hindsight, it was clear that the patient satisfaction pain measure was potentially encouraging physicians to prescribe opioids more than what was necessary. The measure was later removed from the CMS program due to concerns of unintended consequences.

There are several rating programs that are designed to score hospitals and physicians based on their overall care. These programs, such as the Merit-Based Incentive Payment System (MIPS), HVBP program, CMS Overall Star Ratings program, U.S. News and World Report, Leap Frog

Hospital Ratings, and the Premier 100 Top Hospitals program, are all designed to measure a hospital's performance across many facets of care, including patient experience, efficiency, quality, and safety. The programs are inherently designed around balancing measures such that a physician or hospital needs to perform well across measures to receive high marks in the program.

Ranking Measure Performance

If the measure being developed is designed to compare performance across facilities or physicians, it is worthwhile to consider potential bias due to physician or hospital volume. The NHSN HAI measures are a great example of potential low-volume bias. HAIs can be rare occurrences whereby observed events (like MRSA infections) are modeled as an observed to expected ratio. In low volume, the problem with this type of measure is that small hospitals are more likely to lead the charts as top performers when ranking facilities. Even though the measures are risk-adjusted through a ratio of observed to expected events, the chances of a zero for a small hospital are much higher than a large hospital, and so small hospitals generally perform better in the O/E rankings simply due to volume alone. The AHRQ PSI measures are designed to address this problem with the use of a weighted average of hospital performance with a national rate. When we have less volume (or less reliable data) from smaller hospitals, the weight in the weighted average moves their performance toward the national population (due to uncertainty); however, with greater volume (more reliability), the hospital performance weight in the weighted average is small, and the hospital performance is less influenced by the national rate. This also has its challenges, as small hospitals will struggle to achieve a high placement in the rankings when their performance is represented mainly by the national average. One practical solution in these scenarios is to stratify hospitals by a volume measure, such as the number of beds in the facility or the total number of discharges.

Additional Resources

CMS MIPS Measures. https://qpp.cms.gov/mips/explore-measures
Joint Commission Measures. https://www.jointcommission.org/measurement/measures/
CMS Quality Measures. https://www.cms.gov/medicare/quality/initiatives/hospital-quality-initiative

NHSN Measures. https://www.cdc.gov/nhsn/hai-checklists/index.html
AHRQ Measures. https://qualityindicators.ahrq.gov/measures/qi_resources
Care Compare Measure Database. https://data.cms.gov/provider-data/
AHRQ Clinical Classification Software Refined (CCSR). https://hcup-us.ahrq.gov/
    toolssoftware/ccsr/ccs_refined.jsp
UML   Meta-thesaurus.   https://www.nlm.nih.gov/research/umls/knowledge_
    sources/metathesaurus/index.html

3

Hypothesis Testing

To introduce hypothesis testing, let's start with an example. You're a data analyst for a large acute care hospital and have been tasked with measuring the monthly incidence (occurrences) of healthcare-acquired infections (HAIs). In that analysis, you begin with some simple trended reports and observe that, of the various HAIs being evaluated, surgical site infections (SSIs) increased from 1% in September to 3.25% in October of the current year!

You must decide if the shift in SSIs is significant and recommend to the chief quality officer if SSIs should be prioritized above other quality initiatives in the hospital.

You show the preliminary analysis to a few coworkers for their opinions and receive conflicting advice on what recommendation to make. Some coworkers argue that SSIs are uncommon and largely chance events and that you should not read too much into the September to October increase. Others emphasize the severity of SSIs and suggest considering a more rigorous SSI quality improvement initiative.

Resources are limited in the hospital, and you want to make a recommendation that best uses those resources. You ask one more coworker, who happens to have a statistics background, and she recommends a "two-sample test for proportions" to determine if the shift in SSIs is significant. With her help, you conduct the test using a few lines of code and conclude that, given the number of cases of data being evaluated and the variance in the data, the shift is statistically significant and, as a result, recommend that a quality improvement initiative be considered. The question that we have been able to address, with the help of hypothesis testing, is that the shift in SSIs from September to October is not likely to occur by chance and that there is sufficient evidence to indicate a sudden drop in quality of care.

Questions such as these occur frequently in healthcare. You might find that a hospital is spending three dollars more per butterfly needle compared to other hospitals in their health system and need to determine if this cost difference is meaningful. Perhaps you notice that the number of patients receiving

DOI: 10.1201/9781003609759-3

the flu vaccination in October has decreased relative to the prior year. You might observe that the average length of stay for AMI patients is reduced by approximately one day when a newly approved medication is administered, and you want to know if the shift is meaningful. These are all research questions that can be tested with hypothesis testing!

Introduction to Hypothesis Testing

Hypothesis testing is a foundational framework used across a myriad of healthcare disciplines to provide a consistent data-driven method for objective decision-making. The framework gracefully accounts for natural error due to sample size and variance in the data distribution. Through hypothesis testing, we can determine if differences in the data are "statistically significant" within some predefined level of confidence. Without hypothesis testing, the onus is on the individual to subjectively assess whether the observed difference between two quantities is significant.

The term "Hypothesis Testing" can be intimidating and, for some, is reserved solely for formalized experiments conducted by scientists in white lab coats. I'll stress that hypothesis testing should be integral to day-to-day analyses. Seemingly large differences in some supply costs may be insignificant, and seemingly minor differences in inpatient mortality may be highly significant. Without understanding the underlying characteristics of the data being evaluated, we risk acting on meaningless differences or failing to act on a meaningful difference in the data.

Including measures of statistical significance in presentations, technical documentation, and white papers provides additional credibility to your analysis in a consistent and data-driven way. It allows analysts to speak a common language regarding the research question, the level of evidence collected, and the conclusions made through the analyses. Materials that are qualified with measures of statistical significance signal to the stakeholder that the methods are grounded in a robust objective evaluation framework.

Steps to Conduct a Hypothesis Test

We can break down the process of hypothesis testing into a series of steps: (1) define the hypothesis, (2) set the significance level, (3) calculate the test statistic, (4) calculate the *p*-value, and (5) make a decision. Let's work through these steps one by one.

1. Define our hypothesis: With hypothesis testing, we start with two opposing statements—a *null hypothesis* and an *alternate hypothesis*. The null hypothesis assumes the status quo; no difference exists between the two values being compared. Conversely, the alternate hypothesis asserts that there is a statistically significant difference between the evaluated quantities within some predetermined level of confidence. The alternate hypothesis is generally our actual research question; however, we cannot directly prove that an alternate hypothesis is true. We must instead state that, based on the evidence in the data, it is unlikely that the difference is simply a result of chance in the data. In other words, we can say that there is sufficient evidence to reject our null hypothesis with some degree of confidence in favor of our alternate hypothesis.

   I know that this all sounds very noncommittal. In fact, there is a saying about statisticians, "Statistics is the art of never having to say you're wrong". This approach does seem strange at first, but hang in there with me a bit longer, and perhaps you'll agree. With more evidence, you might reject your null hypothesis!

   There are three primary research questions for which we would use hypothesis testing. We might want to know if some quantity of interest (e.g., the proportion of SSIs for September) is *greater* than some comparison or "null" value (e.g., the proportion of SSIs for October). Conversely, we might want to know if the quantity of interest is less than some comparison value. Finally, we might want to know if the quantities are significantly different (in either direction).

   These scenarios are the basis for the left-tailed, right-tailed, and two-tailed tests. Let's pause for a moment and formalize our definitions:

With hypothesis testing, we must distinguish a mean or proportion calculated from a population (i.e., all observations) from a mean or proportion from a sample (i.e., a subset of a population). Samples are error-prone and inherently different from the true value known through the full dataset or population. We will refer to means and proportions from a sample as a "sample statistic" and a mean or proportion calculated from a population as a "parameter". Trust me, without using these terms, you will quickly become annoyed with me spelling out "sample mean or proportion" or "population mean or proportion". Note also that the term test statistic will be used in the subsequent chapters. Be on the lookout for this term as a test statistic and a sample statistic are different concepts that should not be confused with each other. In short, a statistic is calculated from a sample, while a parameter is calculated from the full study population.

Okay, back to the topic at hand—the null and alternate hypotheses.

Null Hypothesis: The null hypothesis asserts that there is no difference between the values being compared—the status quo. In notation, it is typically represented as H_0.

Alternate Hypothesis: Conversely, the alternate hypothesis states that there is a difference between the tested values represented in notation as H_a. The alternate hypothesis generally takes one of three forms: left-tailed, right-tailed, and two-tailed.

> Left-tailed: Testing if the value of interest less than the comparator value.

> Right-tailed: Testing if the value of interest greater than the comparator value.

> Two-tailed: Testing if the value of interest different than the comparator value in either direction.

The full notation for hypothesis testing will vary depending on the characteristics of the data and the research question (e.g., means or proportions). We'll cover these differences later in this chapter, but staying with our SSI example using proportions, we might represent our hypotheses as follows:

- Null Hypothesis (H_0): $p_1 = p_2$
- Alternate Hypothesis: (H_a): $p_1 > p_2$

where p_1 represents the proportion of SSIs from October and p_2 represents the proportion of SSIs from September. We are using a right-tailed test in this example as we are asserting that the proportion of SSIs in October is greater than that of SSIs in September, and therefore, we are using the greater-than symbol in our alternate hypothesis $p_1 > p_2$. If we were to postulate that the proportion of SSIs dropped in October, we could frame the alternate hypothesis of a left-tailed test as $p_1 < p_2$ and, if we were simply interested if the two values were different, we could frame the alternate hypothesis statement of a two-tailed test as $p_1 \neq p_2$.

2. Set the Significance Level: In the first step, it was mentioned that sufficient evidence must exist to reject our null hypothesis in favor of the alternate hypothesis. In this step, we must decide how much evidence will be required (or how confident we must be) to reject our null hypothesis. This value, often called the significance level or alpha α, quantifies the acceptable probability of making an incorrect decision. We can also express our threshold as a "confidence level" $(1-\alpha)$. A .05 (or 5%) significance level, for example, could therefore be rephrased as a .95 (or 95%) confidence level. The most common significance levels are $\alpha = .05$ or $\alpha = .01$, meaning that when we reject the null hypothesis, we are 95% or 99% confident that we have not made an error simply by chance. The choice of a significance level (alpha) might be larger or smaller than the typical values of .05 and .01, depending on the needs of the research question.

3. Calculate the test statistic: A test statistic in hypothesis testing is a numerical value calculated from sample data to assess the strength of evidence against a null hypothesis. It quantifies the difference between the sample data and what would be expected under the null hypothesis. This test statistic is compared to the predefined significance level to determine whether the results are statistically significant, leading to the acceptance or rejection of the null hypothesis.

Depending on the type of hypothesis test, the test statistic will follow different distributions. Commonly used test statistics include t-statistics, z-statistics, chi-square statistics, and F-statistics, which indicate the distribution the statistic follows.

A generalized equation to calculate a test statistic can be expressed as follows:

$$test statistic = \frac{sample statistic - null value}{standard error}$$

where

The sample statistic represents the mean or proportion of the sample data.

The null value represents the comparison value that we will compare our sample statistic against to determine if there is a statistically significant difference between the two values. The null value can be another sample statistic or parameter.

The "standard error" is the sampling statistic's standard deviation.

Standard error is an important concept, so let's spend some time talking about it.

Let us suppose that we sampled 30 inpatient hospitalizations 100 times. For each sample of 30 patients, we calculated the mean length of stay and plotted the distribution of those means as a histogram, as in Figure 3.1.

With each sample, there is the possibility that we happen to select a subset of patients with generally higher or lower mean length of stay values by chance alone. Nothing is materially different about the true mean length of stay we estimate through the sample. We define the standard deviation of these means as the standard error (not deviation). As the size of our sample increases, the degree of variability in the distribution decreases (since the sample becomes more representative of the whole). Conversely, we can expect the standard error to increase with fewer samples, as there is more volatility in the mean with smaller samples.

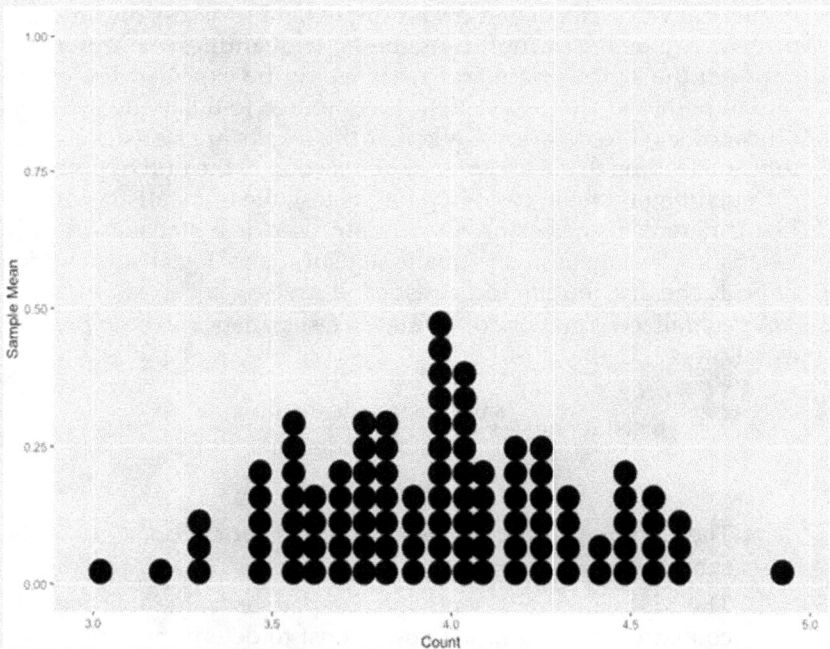

FIGURE 3.1
Histogram showing the normal distribution of mean values derived from 100 samples, each comprised of 30 observations.

We've used an example with means in this case; however, sampling error with proportion data works in a similar way. If we were to sample data using proportions, the number of "successes" in the sample would vary based on the luck of the draw. If we were to plot the distribution of repeated samples of proportion data, we would also end up with a sampling distribution that approaches normal with an increased number of samples. The difference is that the number of "successes" out of "trials" is plotted in the histogram rather than the means of the sample.

Fun fact: In the case of continuous data, even if the underlying data distribution is skewed, the sampling distribution becomes closer to normal, and hypothesis testing is, therefore, fairly resilient to assumptions about normality.

In the paragraphs below, we'll discuss how standard error is calculated, specifically for the type of data and the research question being asked.

Putting it all together, the test statistic measures the standardized difference between the sample statistic and the null value.

4. Calculate the *p*-value: The *p*-value represents the area under the curve outside of the test statistic, which is expressed as a probability; that is, it is the probability of observing a difference as extreme as the one in the sample, assuming the null hypothesis is true.

   That is a confusing sentence, so let's pause for a moment and break this down in simpler terms. We'll use our SSI example for context.

   As shown in Figure 3.2, the area under the curve to the right of the test statistic ($z = 2.3$) corresponds to the probability of obtaining a value as extreme as or even more extreme than our calculated test statistic. In this case, a *z*-score of 2.3 is equivalent to a *p*-value = .01 or 1% (indicating a 1% chance that a proportion of this size would be drawn by chance under the assumption that the null hypothesis is true). A large *p*-value indicates that the differences between the sample statistic and the value expected under the null hypothesis would not be uncommon based on the characteristics of the data. On the other hand, a small *p*-value indicates that the differences in the data are not likely to occur by chance.

   The *p*-value and test statistic provide similar information; however, the *p*-value simply provides a more interpretable value by quantifying the area outside the test statistic relative to the area inside the test statistic. It allows us to say that a test statistic of $z = 2.3$ is equivalent to a 1% chance or less that the sample proportion would be drawn by chance (if our null hypothesis is true).

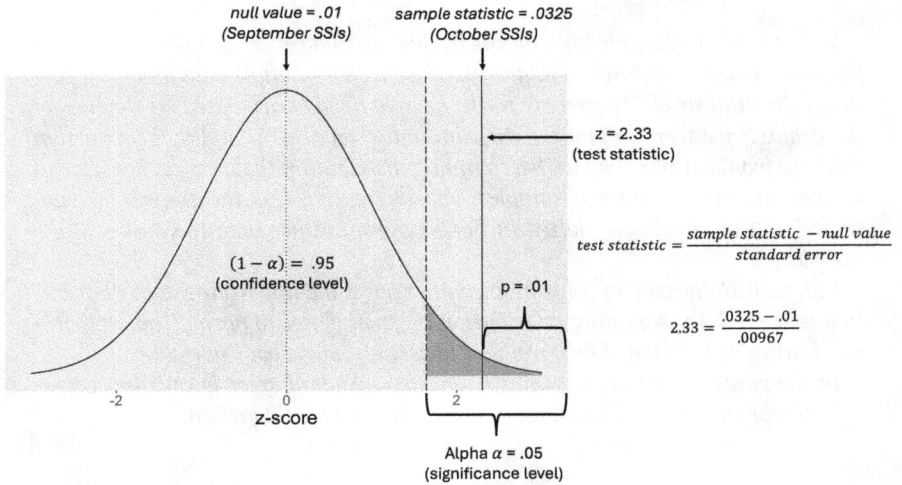

FIGURE 3.2
Normal curve with labeled components used within a hypothesis test using the *p*-value and rejection region methods.

A small *p*-value further indicates stronger evidence for rejecting our null hypothesis (which states that there is no difference in complication proportions from September to October) in favor of our alternate hypothesis (there is a difference in complication proportions from September to October).

When we have small sample sizes and highly variable data, the probability of larger differences in values being compared will be naturally higher, even when no significant difference exists.

We'll talk about how to tactically obtain a *p*-value from a test statistic later in this chapter.

5. Make a decision: Now, you might be asking yourself, at what point have we collected enough evidence to reject our null hypothesis in favor of our alternate hypothesis? In short, we need to compare the evidence gathered from our test (the *p*-value) to the predetermined evidence threshold that we require (alpha or α). If our *p*-value is less than our threshold, we have gathered the evidence needed to reject the null hypothesis in favor of our alternate hypothesis.

In our SSI example, if we set a significance level (α) of .05 before our test and computed a *p*-value of 0.01, we would reject the null hypothesis that the proportion of SSIs from September to October is the same in favor of our alternate hypothesis stating that the proportion of SSIs in October is greater than the proportion of SSIs in September, at a 95% confidence level.

Types of Hypothesis Tests

While the steps to conduct a hypothesis test remain the same, tactically, the types of tests that we employ will vary depending on the nature of the evaluated data. In this section, we'll discuss some of the more commonly used statistical tests. Throughout the remainder of this book, additional statistical tests will be discussed within the context of the chapter topic.

One-Tailed Versus Two-Tailed Tests

Since a two-tailed test is multi-directional, alpha is split between the two tails of the distribution. As demonstrated in Figure 3.3, if we were to set alpha as .05 in a left- or right-tailed test, alpha represents 5% of the data on the left and right tail of the distribution (the area where we will reject the null hypothesis if the test statistic falls within it). However, since a two-tailed test is multi-directional, alpha is split between the two tails, resulting in only 2.5% of the data being segmented at the two tails.

It is important, therefore, to select the appropriate direction for a hypothesis test, as a test statistic may fall outside of alpha in a right-tailed test (e.g.) but may not fall outside of alpha in a two-tailed test. In other words, more evidence is required to reject a null hypothesis in a two-tailed test.

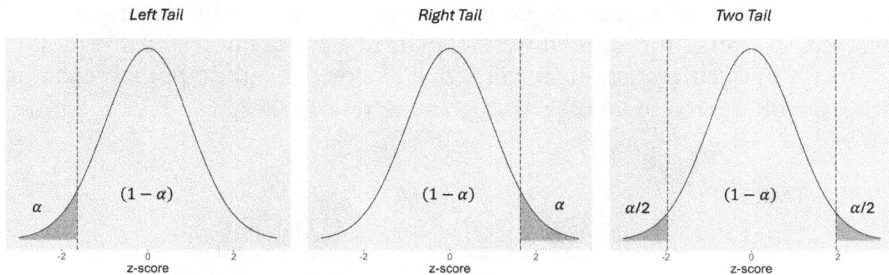

FIGURE 3.3
Alpha thresholds within a normal distribution for left-, right-, and two-tailed hypothesis tests.

Understanding Errors in Hypothesis Testing

In a nutshell, hypothesis testing is the process of clearly stating our research question or business problem in the form of two opposing hypothesis statements, setting a minimum threshold of required evidence and then evaluating the data to determine if the collected evidence is sufficient to assert that the difference is not likely to occur by chance (and therefore statistically significant).

Given that the whole framework of hypothesis testing is based on some level of confidence, mistakes will undoubtedly be made. Note the use of the passive voice to shield myself from any culpability. After all, a 95% confidence level means that, on average, five out of 100 tests (or 1 out of 20) will result in an incorrect conclusion.

There are two ways to draw the wrong conclusions in hypothesis testing. The first is when we incorrectly determine that there is a statistically significant difference in the data (i.e., we reject our null hypothesis) when no actual difference exists. This is referred to as a *Type I error*. In our SSI example, a Type I error would mean that we've incorrectly identified a difference between September and October complications by rejecting our null hypothesis in favor of our alternate hypothesis.

Conversely, we could also fail to detect a significant difference. In this scenario, the difference between September and October SSIs is significant, but our test fails to produce sufficient evidence to reject the null hypothesis at the required evidence threshold (alpha). When we fail to identify a true difference in the data, we have made a *Type II* error.

Just as there are two ways to be wrong, there are also two ways to be right! We can correctly reject our null hypothesis in favor of the alternate hypothesis. Here, the SSI proportions are truly different between the two months, and our test correctly identifies that difference.

We can also correctly conclude that the data has insufficient evidence to reject our null hypothesis. We could correctly state that there is no statistically significant difference in SSI proportions, as shown by the insufficient evidence collected through our test statistic relative to our alpha threshold.

The types of correct and incorrect conclusions through hypothesis testing are often illustrated in tabular form, as shown in Table 3.1.

TABLE 3.1

Type I and Type II Errors in the Hypothesis Testing Process

Test Decision	Reality: Null Hypothesis Is True (No Difference)	Reality: Null Hypothesis Is False
Reject Null Hypothesis	Type I Error	Correct Decision
Accept Null Hypothesis	Correct Decision	Type II Error

THE REJECTION REGION APPROACH
TO HYPOTHESIS TESTING

There are two standard methods for conducting hypothesis testing. We've discussed the "p-value method", in which the p-value derived from the test statistic is compared to the predetermined significance level alpha to assess whether the null hypothesis can be rejected. The second method is the "critical value method", which defines a critical value rather than an alpha before testing.

The critical value sets an evidence threshold based on the sampling distribution (similar to the alpha significance level). For example, for a normal distribution, the critical value would be the z-score representing the boundary where 95% of the data is under the curve, assuming alpha = .05. The region outside the critical value is considered the rejection region.

In this approach, we still calculate a test statistic; however, we do not need to convert the test statistic to a p-value. If the test statistic falls within the rejection region (the area outside of the critical value), we can reject the null hypothesis. This approach is more direct from a computation perspective, but I personally prefer the p-value approach from a conceptual standpoint. This is a matter of personal preference, but I am 75% confident that the p-value method is more interpretable than the critical value method. A visualization showing the relationship between the p-value method and the rejection region method is provided in Figure 3.2.

One Sample Versus Two Sample Hypothesis Testing

Hypothesis tests are generally categorized into two groups: one-sample and two-sample tests. Let's explain these by way of example.

In our working example comparing the proportion of SSIs between September and October, we are dealing with two independent samples. In this scenario, a *two-sample hypothesis test* would be appropriate. We are working with two distinct sets of hospitalizations without overlap and are hypothesizing that there is an increase in the proportion of complications between the two samples (alternate hypothesis).

Let us say that we are now interested in comparing the proportion of SSI complications in September to the proportion of SSIs for the entire year. Here, we have September as a sample, or subset, of all hospitalizations for the year. A scenario like this would call for a *one-sample hypothesis test*, as the sample is a subset of data from the larger population. It should be noted that we don't always know the population value, so this value can be known or hypothesized in a one-sample test.

There is a third scenario where we assess the difference between multiple samples. For example, we might want to know if there is a difference between the SSI proportion across September, October, and November. We will touch on the methods for this type of testing, but for brevity, we will focus on one- and two-sample testing.

Hypothesis Testing for Proportions, Means, and Categorical Variables

Now that we have a conceptual understanding of hypothesis testing, let's practice with some hands-on examples.

Once we have determined if a one-, two-, or multiple-sample test is required, we need to select an appropriate test based on the types of data we are working with.

I know that is a lot of information to process, but don't worry. We'll provide plenty of healthcare-related examples. A set of reference tables has also been included in this chapter, where the hypothesis testing steps using statistical notation are shown side by side with a reproducible example in Python and R. Additionally, a quick reference flowchart to help understand the most appropriate test given the research question and data characteristics is provided in Figure 3.4. We'll use the flow chart to work through examples of each test type. There are some caveats, of course, and it is important to read the fine print after working through the most common scenarios.

We'll begin by evaluating z-tests (and t-tests by extension) for means and proportions.

One-Sample Test for Means

When our goal is to determine if a sample mean (statistic) is different from a population mean (parameter), we can use a one-sample test for means. Depending on the information about the population and the number of observations we are sampling, we will employ either a z-test or t-test. We'll start with the z-test.

z-test

The chief quality officer of a large health system suspects that the patients within their system are generally more acute than average. If she can show

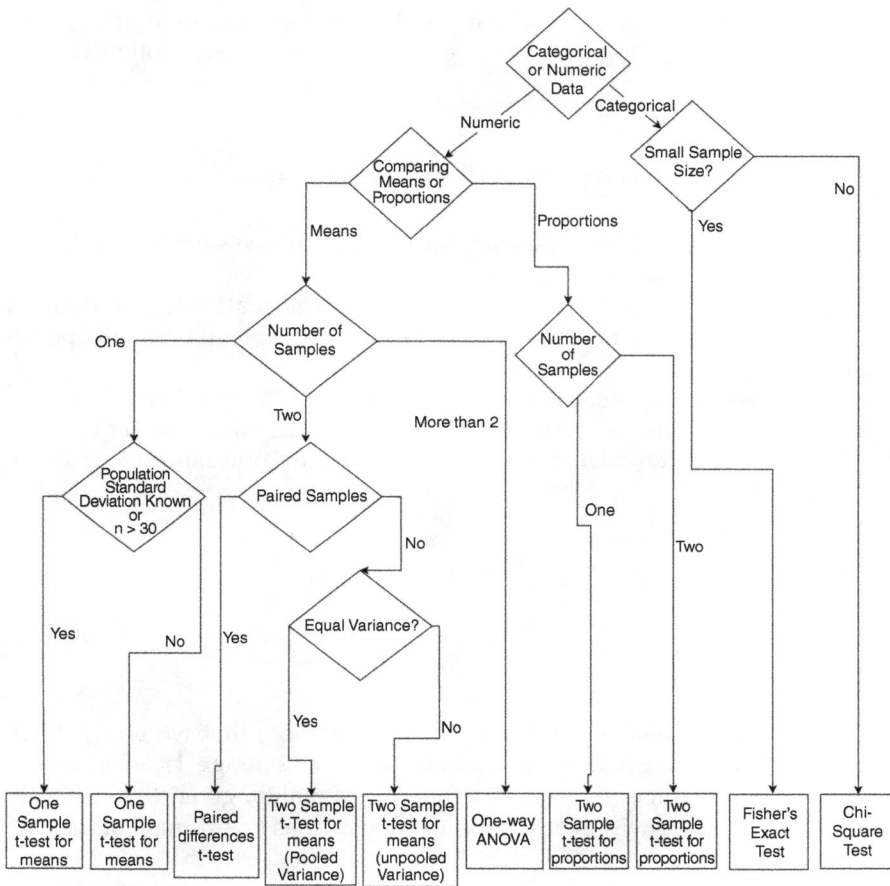

FIGURE 3.4
Flowchart to identify an appropriate hypothesis test.

that their patients are usually more complex, it might help explain the pattern of overall higher rates of morbidity and mortality within their system. One way to approach this problem is to compare the health system's mean case mix index (CMI) to the national CMI average using hypothesis testing. As mentioned in Chapter 2, CMI is an aggregation of hospitalization Medicare Severity Diagnosis Related Group (MS-DRG) weights that drive hospital Medicare reimbursement; however, it is often used as a proxy for patient complexity (under the assumption that high-cost patients are generally more acute).

In forming our hypothesis statement, we must listen carefully to the business problem. Since the Chief Quality Officer (CQO) is asking if the mean

CMI is higher than average (and not simply that they are different), a right-tailed test is more appropriate. We'll set up our hypotheses as follows:

$$\text{NullHypothesis}(H_0): \mu = \mu_0$$

$$\text{AlternateHypothesis}(H_a): \mu > \mu_0$$

where μ is the mean CMI for the health system (sample statistic), and μ_0 is the national CMI (parameter) across all U.S. hospitals.

We can see that our alternate hypothesis $\mu > \mu_0$ (the real motivation behind our analysis) asserts that the health system mean μ is greater than the population mean μ_0.

We'll also set our significance level as $\alpha = .05$ (a 95% confidence level).

Now that we've formed our hypothesis statement and have set our significance level, we can calculate our z-statistic using a one-sample z-test. The z-test takes the following form:

$$z = \frac{\bar{x} - \mu_0}{\dfrac{\sigma}{\sqrt{n}}}$$

where

- $\bar{x}$ is the health system CMI being evaluated. Note that we use $\bar{x}$ (pronounced "x bar") here to indicate that the average is an estimate. The true average μ cannot be known in reality, given the naturally occurring error within any sample. We use $\bar{x}$ as an estimate of the true mean μ.

- μ_0 is the national CMI (the hypothesized value) across all national hospitals. Our null hypothesis asserts that the health system CMI μ (estimated by $\bar{x}$) is equal to the national CMI μ_0.

- $\dfrac{\sigma}{\sqrt{n}}$ is the standard error, which is formed by the known standard deviation σ of all hospital CMI values (i.e., the population) divided by the square root of the total number of hospitals n in our sample (the health system).

- z is the test statistic indicating the number of standardized units away from the hypothesized value μ_0

Recall that the area under the curve to the right of the test statistic corresponds to the probability of obtaining a value as extreme or more extreme than the test statistic.

We can represent the *p*-value from our test statistic as follows:

$$p = P(Z \geq z)$$

where

z is our test statistic (a z-score in this case).

Z represents a random variable.

p is the *p*-value obtained from the test statistic.

we can, therefore, interpret $p = P(Z \geq z)$ as the probability that some random variable Z is greater than the test statistic z. In other words, it is the area under the curve to the right of the test statistic.

Note that if we were conducting a left-tailed test, the p-value would be represented as $P(Z \leq z)$ and the p-value for a two-tailed test as $p = 2 \times P(Z \geq |z|)$. The multiplication by 2 is specifically used in a two-tailed test to account for both tails of the distribution. Since a two-tailed test considers extreme values in both the positive and negative directions, we need to consider both sides of the distribution to calculate the p-value.

If the *p*-value is less than alpha α, we reject the null hypothesis in favor of the alternate hypothesis.

Enough muddling around with notation. Let's look at an implementation of a one-sample test for means using Python.

```
import numpy as np
from scipy.stats import norm
health_system_cmi = np.array([1.02, 1.1, 1.05, 0.95,
0.98, 0.92, 1.12, 1.01, 1.05, 0.93])
national_mean_cmi = 1.0
population_std = 0.1
alpha = 0.05
sample_mean = np.mean(health_system_cmi)
n = len(health_system_cmi)
z_score = (sample_mean - national_mean_cmi) /
(population_std / np.sqrt(n))
p_value = 1 - norm.cdf(z_score)
if p_value < alpha:
```

```
    print("There is sufficient evidence to suggest that
the health system's mean CMI is greater than the national
mean CMI.")
else:
    print("There is insufficient evidence to suggest that
the health system's mean CMI is greater than the national
mean CMI.")
```

In this Python example, we have an array `health_system_cmi` containing CMI values within the health system being evaluated, as well as the hypothesized value `national_mean_cmi`. We then compute a standard error (`population_std` / `np.sqrt(n)`) using the known population standard deviation (`population_std`) to produce the `z-statistic`. The `norm.cdf` function from `scipy.stats` calculates the cumulative distribution function (CDF) of the standard normal distribution and obtains the right-tailed *p*-value. In other words, it computes the area under the curve within (to the left of) the test statistic. We then determine if the *p*-value obtained from the test statistic is less than alpha. If so, we will reject the null hypothesis in favor of the alternate hypothesis.

An implementation in R will resemble the Python implementation above:

```
health_system_cmi <- c(1.02, 1.1, 1.05, 0.95, 0.98, 0.92,
1.12, 1.01, 1.05, 0.93)
national_mean_cmi <- 1.0
population_std <- 0.1
alpha <- 0.05

sample_mean <- mean(health_system_cmi)
n <- length(health_system_cmi)

z_score <- (sample_mean - national_mean_cmi) /
(population_std / sqrt(n))
p_value <- 1 - pnorm(z_score)

if (p_value < alpha) {
  print("There is sufficient evidence to suggest that the
health system's mean CMI is greater than the national
mean CMI.")
} else {
  print("There is insufficient evidence to suggest that
the health system's mean CMI is greater than the national
mean CMI.")
}
```

Using R, we similarly have a vector `health_system_cmi` containing CMI values as well as the hypothesized value `national_mean_cmi`. We also compute a standard error (`population_std` / `sqrt(n)`) using the known population standard deviation (`population_std`) to produce the z-statistic. The `pnorm` function calculates the CDF of the standard normal distribution and obtains the right-tailed *p*-value. We then determine if the *p*-value obtained from the test statistic is less than `alpha` to either reject or fail to reject our null hypothesis.

t-test

As discussed in the previous section, to conduct a z-test, we must have access to the population standard deviation σ. In the CMI example above, we have access to the publicly available data for all hospitals (the population) and, therefore, have the luxury of a z-test. When the population standard deviation is unknown, we can use the sample standard deviation s in its place to estimate the population standard deviation as part of a "Student's t-test". In the CMI example, this would be the standard deviation of the CMI values within the health system being evaluated. The t-test, therefore, takes the following form:

$$t = \frac{\bar{x} - \mu_0}{\frac{s}{\sqrt{n}}}$$

where

- $\bar{x}$ is the health system mean being evaluated (as an estimate of the true system mean μ).
- μ_0 is the national health system mean (the hypothesized value).
- $\frac{s}{\sqrt{n}}$ is the standard error, which is formed by the estimated standard deviation s of health system CMI values (i.e., the sample) divided by the square root of the total count of hospitals n in our sample (the health system).

The t-test is a more conservative test used when the population standard deviation is unknown (and, therefore, must be estimated through the sample standard deviation, not the population standard deviation). It is also common for the t-test to be employed when the sample size is small. The t-distribution is parameterized by the sample size n (technically, the degrees of freedom, which is n-1), allowing the distribution to change shape based on the number of samples—requiring more evidence with small sample sizes. We will use software to calculate the *p*-value; however, in the days of old, statisticians would look up *p*-values based on the sample size and test statistic.

The results of the z-test and t-test will largely converge as the sample size increases.

A Python implementation of a one-sample t-test for means using our CMI use-case is as follows:

```python
import numpy as np
from scipy.stats import ttest_1samp
health_system_cmi = np.array([1.02, 1.1, 1.05, 0.95,
0.98, 0.92, 1.12, 1.01, 1.05, 0.93])
national_mean_cmi = 1.0
alpha = 0.05
test_statistic, p_value = ttest_1samp(health_system_cmi,
national_mean_cmi, alternative='greater')
if p_value < alpha:
    print("There is sufficient evidence to suggest that
the health system's mean CMI is greater than the national
mean CMI.")
else:
    print("There is insufficient evidence to suggest that
the health system's mean CMI is greater than the national
mean CMI.")
```

The test statistic for a one-sample t-test for means can be calculated using the `ttest_1samp` function from the `scipy.stats` subpackage—which abstracts away the pesky p-value calculation from the t-statistic. This function returns test statistic and p-value when provided the sample statistic `health_system_cmi` and hypothesized value `national_mean_cmi` and test direction `alternative='greater'`:

```python
ttest_1samp(health_system_cmi, national_mean_cmi,
alternative='greater')
```

In R, the t.test function calculates the t-statistic for us, with similar arguments for the sample vector, population mean, and the "alternative".

```r
health_system_cmi <- c(1.02, 1.1, 1.05, 0.95, 0.98, 0.92,
1.12, 1.01, 1.05, 0.93)
national_mean_cmi <- 1.0
alpha <- 0.05

test_result <- t.test(health_system_cmi, mu = national_
mean_cmi, alternative = "greater")

test_statistic <- test_result$statistic
p_value <- test_result$p.value

if (p_value < alpha) {
```

```
   print("There is sufficient evidence to suggest that the
health system's mean CMI is greater than the national
mean CMI.")
} else {
   print("There is insufficient evidence to suggest that
the health system's mean CMI is greater than the national
mean CMI.")
}
```

Example implementations for the one-sample left-, right-, and two-tailed z-tests and t-tests means are provided in Tables 3.5–3.11.

Two-Sample Test for Means

In the one-sample test for means, a sample is compared to the larger population to determine if there is a statistically significant difference between the sample and population mean. Another scenario that we commonly encounter is the need to compare two independent samples. Perhaps a health system recently acquired another health system (an increasingly common occurrence), and the CQO now wants to know if the hospital CMI values for the acquiring health system are different on average from those in the acquired health system. In other words, is the overall risk profile for patients in their health system different from those in the health system being acquired? The distribution of CMI values are independent samples without overlap, making the two-sample test for means a suitable choice. Furthermore, a two-tailed test is appropriate since the objective is to measure the difference in either direction.

We'll set up our hypotheses as follows:

$$\text{NullHypothesis}(H_0): \mu_1 - \mu_2 = 0$$

$$\text{AlternateHypothesis}(H_a): \mu_1 - \mu_2 \neq 0$$

where μ_1 and μ_2 are the sample CMI means for the two health systems being evaluated.

While we use a two-tailed test in this example, a left- and right-tailed test would be represented as $\mu_1 - \mu_2 > 0$ and $\mu_1 - \mu_2 < 0$, respectively (indicating the direction of the difference).

The null hypothesis in the two-sample test asserts that there is no difference between the two CMI distributions, while our alternate hypothesis states that there is a difference (within some level of confidence).

We'll use a significance level of $\alpha = .05$ (or a 95% confidence level).

In the two-sample test, each sample will have its own variance. If the variance is the same, we can use "pooled variance" s_p where the variance is weighted by the number of observations in the two samples. Otherwise, a test using unpooled variance should be employed. As a rough test, if the ratio of variances between the two samples is between 0.5 and 2, we can say that the variance is roughly equal (one is less than double the other). If needed, more formalized tests exist to determine equal variance, such as the F-test for equal variance.

Let's look at a two-sample t-test for comparing means using unpooled variance:

$$t = \frac{\bar{x}_1 - \bar{x}_2 - 0}{\sqrt{\dfrac{s_1^2}{n_1} + \dfrac{s_2^2}{n_2}}}$$

Note that we will not show a z-test as it is rare for both population standard deviations to be known. This said that the one-sample z-test and t-test are analogous to the two-sample z-test and t-test. One can simply replace the sample standard deviations s with the population standard deviation σ to obtain the test statistic. Remember that the z- and t-tests follow different distributions (with the latter conditioned on sample size).

When variance is roughly equal, the variance can be pooled.

$$t = \frac{\bar{x}_1 - \bar{x}_2 - 0}{s_p \sqrt{\dfrac{1}{n_1} + \dfrac{1}{n_2}}}$$

$$s_p = \sqrt{\frac{(n_1 - 1)s_1^2 + (n_2 - 1)s_2^2}{n_1 + n_2 - 2}}$$

where s_p is the pooled (or combined) variance between the two samples.

In the following, we have an implementation of the CMI research question using Python. In this example, we use the `ttest_ind` function from `scipy.stats` to conduct the two-sample test for means. This test pools the variance with the `equal_var` argument set to `True`. Consistent with the previous example, we will use a two-tailed test. To use unpooled variance, the `equal_var` argument would be set to `False`.

```
import numpy as np
from scipy.stats import ttest_ind
```

```
health_system_a = np.array([1.93, 1.53, 1.18, 2.09,
1.68])
health_system_b = np.array([1.63, 0.97, 1.93, 2.02,
1.46])

t_statistic, p_value = ttest_ind(health_system_a, health_
system_b, alternative='two-sided',equal_var=True) #set
equal_var=False for unpooled

alpha = 0.05

if p_value < alpha:
    print("There is sufficient evidence to reject the
null hypothesis in favor of the alternate hypothesis.")
else:
    print("There is insufficient evidence to reject the
null hypothesis.")
```

Using R, we can pull the variance in an similar manner using the native t.test function:

```
health_system_a <- c(1.93, 1.53, 1.18, 2.09, 1.68)
health_system_b <- c(1.63, 0.97, 1.93, 2.02, 1.46)

ttest_result <- t.test(health_system_a, health_system_b,
alternative = "two.sided", var.equal = TRUE) # Set var.
equal = FALSE for unpooled

p_value <- ttest_result$p.value

alpha <- 0.05

if (p_value < alpha) {
  print("There is sufficient evidence to reject the null
hypothesis in favor of the alternate hypothesis.")
} else {
  print("There is insufficient evidence to reject the
null hypothesis.")
}
```

Paired Difference t-test for Means

The paired difference t-test is designed for situations where two measurements are taken from the same subject under different conditions. The main idea is to assess whether there is a statistically significant difference between the sets of paired observations. For example, we might want to compare measurements before treatment to those following treatment. Therefore, each patient would have two measurements, and we want to determine if the mean difference between those measurements is statistically significant.

Hypothesis statements are structured a bit differently with a paired difference test, as we have two sets of data from the same subjects. Our null hypothesis states that there is no difference between the two sets of measurements, while the alternate hypothesis states that there is a statistically significant difference between the matched pairs. Like the previous tests we've discussed, we might be interested in a negative, positive, or overall difference between the two sets of observations, evaluated through left-, right-, and two-tailed tests.

Suppose a researcher is studying a new drug treatment called Reduceamine (pronounced reduce-a-mean), designed to lower blood pressure in hypertensive patients. She wants to determine whether Reduceamine effectively lowers blood pressure within the same group of patients over time.

The researcher selects a group of hypertensive patients and measures their blood pressure before administering the new drug treatment. After a set period, the researcher measures their blood pressure again.

Hypothesis: The null hypothesis (H_0) states that the mean blood pressure is the same before and after administering Reduceamine. The alternative hypothesis (H_a) states that the mean blood pressure decreases after administering Reduceamine.

The researcher records each patient's blood pressure before and after the treatment. This gives us paired data for each individual, representing the difference between the before-treatment and after-treatment measurements.

A paired difference t-test for means is conducted to determine if there is a statistically significant reduction in the mean blood pressure before and after the treatment (a left-tailed test).

$$\text{NullHypothesis}(H_0): \mu_d = 0$$

$$\text{AlternateHypothesis}(H_a): \mu_d < 0$$

where $\bar{d}$ represents the difference between the two values.

$$t = \frac{\bar{d}}{\frac{s_d}{\sqrt{n}}}$$

The alternate hypothesis $\mu_d < 0$ is that of a left-tailed test, where we are asserting that there is a decrease in blood pressure between the two sets of measurements. If we were interested in a two-tailed or right-tailed test, we could represent those alternate hypotheses as $\mu_d \neq 0$ or $\mu_d > 0$.

The standard error, like the one-sample test, is comprised of the standard deviation of the differences over the square root of the number of matched pairs.

Python

```python
import numpy as np
from scipy import stats

before_treatment = np.array([140, 150, 135, 160, 155,
110, 125])
after_treatment = np.array([130, 140, 125, 145, 140, 135,
130])

differences = after_treatment - before_treatment

alpha = 0.05

t_statistic, p_value = stats.ttest_rel(after_treatment,
before_treatment, alternative = 'less')

if p_value < alpha:
    print("Reject the null hypothesis. The treatment has
a significant effect on reducing blood pressure.")
else:
    print("Fail to reject the null hypothesis. There
is no significant effect of the treatment on blood
pressure.")
```

R

```r
before_treatment <- c(140, 150, 135, 160, 155, 110, 125)
after_treatment <- c(130, 140, 125, 145, 140, 135, 130)

differences <- after_treatment - before_treatment

alpha <- 0.05

ttest_result <- t.test(after_treatment, before_treatment,
paired = TRUE, alternative = "less")

p_value <- ttest_result$p.value

if (p_value < alpha) {
  print("Reject the null hypothesis. The treatment has a
significant effect on reducing blood pressure.")
} else {
  print("Fail to reject the null hypothesis. There is no
significant effect of the treatment on blood pressure.")
}
```

One-Sample Test for Proportions

We've discussed various scenarios involving testing two means, but how do we deal with testing data that involves proportions? As detailed in Chapter 2, there is no shortage of proportion measures in healthcare measurement and evaluation. Process and outcome measures are often binary in nature and are ideal candidates for tests about proportions. A process was followed or not, and a complication occurred or did not. Various tests are available for proportions, just as there are for testing means.

Perhaps a family physician is interested in evaluating the control of high blood pressure in her patient population, an HEDIS measure. High blood pressure is a major risk factor for various serious health conditions, including heart disease, stroke, kidney disease, and vascular disorders. Detecting and managing high blood pressure can significantly reduce the risk of developing these conditions.

In accordance with the measure definition, patients 18–85 years of age with a diagnosis of hypertension within the last year will be tested during their office visit. These patients will make up the denominator of our proportion. If the patient's blood pressure is less than 140/90 mm Hg, then the patient's blood pressure will be identified as "adequately controlled" (a numerator value of 1). Otherwise, the patient's blood pressure will be designated as not adequately controlled through a 0 value in the numerator.

Since this is an National Quality Forum (NQF)-endorsed HEDIS measure, the national average is published on the National Committee for Quality Assurance (NCQA) website. For demonstration, we'll use the population proportion of 60.3, indicating that 60.3% of the national population has adequately controlled blood pressure.

The physician wants to assess whether her patients' blood pressure is being managed better or worse relative to the national average. Here, we have a scenario that can be tested using a one-sample test for proportions. That is, we have a sample of a population (e.g., patients visiting the physician's office), and we want to test whether there is a statistically significant difference between the samples p and the hypothesized proportion of patients with high blood pressure p_0.

The null and alternate hypotheses are analogous to the one-sample test for means in that the null hypothesis asserts that the two samples are not different and will reject the null hypothesis in favor of the alternate hypothesis with sufficient evidence. Since the physician is interested in increased measure compliance, we will conduct a right-tailed test.

$$\text{Null Hypothesis } H_0 : p = p_0$$

$$\text{Alternate Hypothesis} (H_a) : p > p_0$$

Just as we used $\bar{x}$ to estimate the true sample mean μ, we used $\hat{p}$ to estimate the true sample proportion p. In our example, $\hat{p}$ represents the proportion of eligible patients whose blood pressure is under control according to the measure definition. The hypothesized value p_0 is the national proportion of patients whose blood pressure is under control. We'll use a one-sample z-test for proportions. For reference, the left- and two-tailed test can be represented as $p < p_0$ and $p \neq p_0$.

To determine the test statistic, we must calculate the standard error. As with the one-sample test for means, the numerator of our test considers the difference in the two sample values, while the denominator is comprised of the standard error. For a one-sample test for proportion, the standard error is calculated as $\sqrt{\dfrac{p_0(1-p_0)}{n}}$ where n represents the number of observations within the sample (i.e., physician office visits).

$$z = \frac{\hat{p} - p_0}{\sqrt{\dfrac{p_0(1-p_0)}{n}}}$$

It should be noted that a t-test for proportions exists, but in practice, the z-test is much more prevalent. To compute the z-statistic and p-value in Python, we can use the proportions_ztest function from the statsmodels.stats.proportion subpackage.

```
import numpy as np
from statsmodels.stats.proportion import
proportions_ztest

bp_under_control = 64
hypertension_pat = 100

null_hypothesis_proportion = .603

alpha = 0.05

z_statistic, p_value = proportions_ztest(bp_under_
control, hypertension_pat, null_hypothesis_proportion)

if p_value < alpha:
    print("Reject the null hypothesis in favor of the
alternate hypothesis.")
else:
    print("Fail to reject the null hypothesis.")
```

Using R, we can use the prop.test function for convenience.

```
bp_under_control <- 64
hypertension_pat <- 100
```

```
null_hypothesis_proportion <- 0.603

alpha <- 0.05

test_result <- prop.test(x = bp_under_control, n =
hypertension_pat, p = null_hypothesis_proportion,
alternative = "greater", correct = FALSE)

p_value <- test_result$p.value

if (p_value < alpha) {
  print("Reject the null hypothesis in favor of the
alternate hypothesis.")
} else {
  print("Fail to reject the null hypothesis.")
}
```

When there isn't enough data to satisfy the assumptions of a one-sample test for proportions, it might be worth considering a test that falls under the category of exact tests or nonparametric tests, such as *Fisher's Exact Test*. These tests do not rely heavily on distributional assumptions and are often used when data is limited or doesn't meet the assumptions of traditional parametric tests.

Two-Sample Test for Proportions

Similar to the two-sample test for means, there are times when we are interested in testing for differences between two independent samples of proportion data. Consistent with the previous tests, the null hypothesis assumes no difference in the proportions, while the alternate hypothesis asserts that there is a statistically significant difference—with an option for a left-, right-, or two-tailed test.

In the section on hypothesis testing, we discussed comparing the proportion of surgical site infections between two time periods. Let's revisit this example. To ensure a sufficient sample size, we will compare the proportion of SSIs in a large hospital's medical/surgical ward between the current and previous years. We are interested in whether the proportion of SSIs this year differs from the previous year. We will conduct a two-tailed test.

$$\text{Null } H_0 : p_1 = p_2$$

$$\text{Alternate } H_a : \text{Two Tail} : p_1 \neq p_2$$

For reference, a left- and right-tailed test would take the form of $p_1 < p_2$ and $p_1 > p_2$, respectively.

To compute the test statistic, we must estimate the standard error of the difference by combining the variance from the two samples $\sqrt{\hat{p}(1-\hat{p})\left(\dfrac{1}{n_1}+\dfrac{1}{n_2}\right)}$.

$$z = \frac{\hat{p}_1 - \hat{p}_2 - 0}{\sqrt{\hat{p}(1-\hat{p})\left(\dfrac{1}{n_1}+\dfrac{1}{n_2}\right)}}$$

$$\hat{p} = \frac{x_1 + x_2}{n_1 + n_2}$$

The pooled sample proportion $\hat{p}$ is the combined proportion of successes from both samples over the total combined sample size, considering the proportions from both groups.

Python

To compute the z-statistic and *p*-value, we can again use the `propor-tions_ztest` function from the `statsmodels.stats.proportion` subpackage.

```
import numpy as np
from statsmodels.stats.proportion import
proportions_ztest
current_year_ssi = 15
current_year_n = 394

previous_year_ssi = 11
previous_year_n = 351

ssi_counts = np.array([current_year_ssi,
previous_year_ssi])
sample_sizes = np.array([current_year_n,
previous_year_n])

alpha = 0.05

z_statistic, p_value = proportions_ztest(ssi_counts,
sample_sizes, alternative = 'larger')

if p_value < alpha:
    print("Reject the null hypothesis in favor of the
alternate hypothesis.")
else:
    print("Fail to reject the null hypothesis.")
```

R

Again we will use the prop.test function in the R implementation.

```
current_year_ssi <- 15
current_year_n <- 394

previous_year_ssi <- 11
previous_year_n <- 351

alpha <- 0.05

test_result <- prop.test(c(current_year_ssi, previous_
year_ssi), c(current_year_n, previous_year_n),
alternative = "greater", correct = FALSE)

p_value <- test_result$p.value

if (p_value < alpha) {
  print("Reject the null hypothesis in favor of the
alternate hypothesis.")
} else {
  print("Fail to reject the null hypothesis.")
}
```

It's important to note that the prop.test function in R has a correct argument, which applies a "continuity correction". This correction helps improve the accuracy of the results by accounting for the slight differences between continuous and discrete distributions, particularly when sample sizes are small, or the proportion is near 0 or 1.

Chi-Square Test

How do we conduct a hypothesis test when comparing categorical data? In most cases, we can employ a chi-square test.

The test involves comparing the observed frequencies in each category of a contingency table with the frequencies expected under the assumption of independence between the variables. The resulting test statistic follows a chi-square distribution.

Let's start with some test data in the form of a 2 × 2 (or "two by two") table showing patient counts for patients with and without a history of bariatric surgery for weight loss, segmented further by those with subsequent development of osteoporosis (Table 3.2).

To begin, we must calculate expected values corresponding to each observed value in the 2 × 2 table. The expected value E is calculated for each row i and column j and is represented as E_{ij}. Specifically, we obtain E_{ij} by dividing the product of the row and column totals by the grand total:

$$E_{ij} = \frac{\text{row total} \times \text{column total}}{\text{grand total}}$$

TABLE 3.2

An Example of a 2 × 2 Contingency Table

Exposure	New Cases (Osteoporosis)	Controls (No Osteoporosis)	Total
Had bariatric surgery	5	40	45
Did not have bariatric surgery	35	3,420	3,455
Total	40	3,460	3,500

TABLE 3.3

Calculations for the Expected Values Used within a Chi-Square Test

Exposure	New Cases (Osteoporosis)	Controls (No Osteoporosis)	Total
Had bariatric surgery	**0.51** = (45 × 40)/3500	**44.49** = (45 ×3,460)/3500	45
Did not have bariatric surgery	**39.49** = (3,455 × 40)/3500	**3,415.51** = (3,455 ×3,460)/3500	3,455
Total	40	3,460	3,500

E_{ij} is therefore an estimate of the expected counts. For demonstration, expected values are calculated using the osteoporosis data from Table 3.2 and are shown in Table 3.3.

The chi-square test evaluates whether there is a significant association between two categorical variables. Now that we have the expected values calculated, we can calculate the chi-square test statistic χ^2 as follows:

$$\chi^2 = \sum \frac{\left(O_{ij} - E_{ij}\right)^2}{E_{ij}}$$

The chi-square statistic is a test statistic similar to a z- or t-statistic discussed in the chapter on hypothesis testing. Rather than a z- or t-distribution, however, we are assuming in this case that the test statistic follows a chi-square distribution. Again, using our working example, we can calculate the chi-square test statistic as follows:

To obtain the chi-square statistic, we simply sum overall cells in the contingency table (Table 3.4).

$$\chi^2 = a + b + c + d$$

Or in our example:

$$\sim 40.49 = 39.53 + 0.45 + 0.51 + .006$$

TABLE 3.4

Calculations of Final Quadrant Values with a Chi-Square Test

Exposure	New Cases (Osteoporosis)	Controls (No Osteoporosis)
Had bariatric surgery	$39.53 = \dfrac{(5 - 0.51)^2}{.51}$	$.45 = \dfrac{(40 - 44.49)^2}{44.49}$
Did not have bariatric surgery	$.51 = \dfrac{(35 - 39.49)^2}{39.49}$	$.006 = \dfrac{(3420 - 3,415.51)^2}{3415.51}$

Like other hypothesis tests, the *p*-value can be obtained with the test statistic and degrees of freedom. Luckily, we have fantastic Python libraries to help us derive the values—in this case, the scipy.stats library.

```
from scipy.stats import chi2_contingency
contingency_table = [[5, 40], [35, 3420]]

chi2, p, dof, expected =
chi2_contingency(contingency_table,correction=False)

print(f"Chi-square Statistic: {chi2:.2f}")
print(f"P-value: {p:.2f}")
print(f"DOF: {dof:.2f}")
print(f"Expected: {expected}")
```

And in R, the chi-square statistic can be calculated with the native chisq. test function.

```
contingency_table <- matrix(c(5, 40, 35, 3420), nrow = 2,
byrow = TRUE)

test_result <- chisq.test(contingency_table, correct =
FALSE)

cat("Chi-square Statistic:", round(test_result$statistic,
2), "\n")
cat("P-value:", round(test_result$p.value, 2), "\n")
cat("Degrees of Freedom:", test_result$parameter, "\n")
cat("Expected Frequencies:\n")
print(test_result$expected)
```

In this implementation, we use the chisq.test function in R to perform a chi-squared test on a contingency table. The matrix function creates the table with nrow = 2 to specify two rows, and byrow = TRUE ensures that the data is entered into the matrix row by row, meaning the first two values form the first row, the next two values form the second row, and so on.

With a *p*-value of <.001, we can reject our null hypothesis stating that there is no association between osteoporosis incidence and bariatric surgery.

Fisher Exact Test

One limitation of the Chi-square test is that it can produce volatile results when counts in any one quadrant are small (where less than 5 or 10). The Fisher exact test is a great alternative that can be used to determine the statistical significance of the association between two categorical variables (e.g., exposure and disease), especially when sample sizes are small. The test calculates the probability of observing a distribution as extreme as, or more extreme than, the observed distribution, given the totals of the table. It is particularly useful for small sample sizes and when exact probabilities are needed, but it may become computationally intensive for larger tables. The nuances of the test are beyond the scope of this book; however, an implementation in Python and R have been provided below:

Python

```
from scipy.stats import fisher_exact
contingency_table = [[5, 40], [35, 3,420]]
odds_ratio, p_value = fisher_exact(contingency_table)
print(f"Odds Ratio: {odds_ratio}")
print(f"P-value: {p_value}")
```

R

```
contingency_table <- matrix(c(5, 40, 35, 3420), nrow = 2,
byrow = TRUE)
test_result <- fisher.test(contingency_table)
cat("Odds Ratio:", test_result$estimate, "\n")
cat("P-value:", test_result$p.value, "\n")
```

Checking Assumptions

We must check our assumptions for all statistical tests to ensure that we're using the test as intended. These are *parametric* tests that are built under the assumption that certain data conditions are present. Incorrect use of the test can lead to erroneous conclusions, ultimately harming the patient or resulting in wasteful care. Some assumptions are firm, while others are flexible, and it is essential to have a firm grasp of these assumptions before selecting the type of test. Assumptions for each test are listed at the top of Tables 3.5–3.11.

When Normality Assumptions Are Violated

In healthcare analysis, hypothesis testing is commonly used to compare patient outcomes, such as length of stay and cost. Hospital administrators might want to know if an operational improvement has reduced the overall length of stay or if switching contracts on a particular supply has resulted in material savings.

A challenge with using length of stay and cost data, as well as similarly distributed data, is that they exhibit a rightward skewed distribution (i.e., the data has a long tail to the right). While hypothesis tests are somewhat resilient to skewed data, we can apply a natural log transformation to mitigate potential bias resulting from skewed data. This correction technique will often coerce the data into a normal distribution, allowing standard z-tests and t-tests to be applied to the data with less concern about normality assumptions.

The test statistic will be computed just as before; however, as a preprocessing step, a log transformation will be applied to the data points (such as a patient's length of stay or cost).

Below is an example of a one-sample t-test for means using log-transformed cost data for CPAP machine values. This distribution is slightly rightward skewed, with some high-cost outliers. A log transformation will mitigate the effect of the extreme values by coercing the distribution closer to normal, satisfying our test assumptions.

Python

```
import numpy as np
import scipy.stats as stats
cpap_cost = np.array([120, 150, 100, 180, 400, 350, 300,
320, 310, 200, 180, 220, 110, 150, 640, 400, 280, 130,
480, 250,
160, 370, 430, 810, 160, 1300, 500, 1230, 400, 140, 220,
1150, 270, 120, 250, 210, 180, 190, 240, 140, 380, 290,
230, 140, 480, 200, 130, 330, 370])

sample_log_cpap_cost = np.log(cpap_cost)
population_log_cpap_mean = np.log(375)

alpha = 0.05
t_statistic, p_value = stats.ttest_1samp(sample_log_cpap_
cost, population_log_cpap_mean, alternative='two-sided')
```

```
if p_value < alpha:
    print("Reject the null hypothesis")
else:
    print("Fail to reject the null hypothesis")
```

R

```
cpap_cost <- c(120, 150, 100, 180, 400, 350, 300, 320,
310, 200, 180, 220, 110, 150, 640, 400, 280, 130, 480,
250,
                160, 370, 430, 810, 160, 1300, 500, 1230,
400, 140, 220, 1150, 270, 120, 250, 210, 180, 190, 240,
                140, 380, 290, 230, 140, 480, 200, 130,
330, 370)

log_cpap_cost <- log(cpap_cost)

population_log_cpap_mean <- log(375)

alpha <- 0.05

test_result <- t.test(log_cpap_cost, mu = population_log_
cpap_mean, alternative = "two.sided")

cat("t-statistic:", round(test_result$statistic, 2),
"\n")
cat("p-value:", round(test_result$p.value, 4), "\n")

if (test_result$p.value < alpha) {
  cat("Reject the null hypothesis\n")
} else {
  cat("Fail to reject the null hypothesis\n")
}
```

For wildly irregular distributions (e.g., multi-modal, extreme skew), other "non-parametric" tests, such as the Mann Wilcoxon Rank-Sum or the Kruskal-Wallis test, can be considered. These tests are outside this book's scope, but it is important to know that there is further recourse when such conditions exist in the data.

Statistical Significance Versus Practical Significance

One criticism of hypothesis testing is that any test will become significant with a large enough sample. Access to large datasets is commonplace today, and it is not unusual to have samples in the thousands, hundreds of thousands, or millions (or more). As the sample size increases, the standard error incrementally shrinks, causing such tests to be highly sensitive to minuscule changes in the means. While such changes may be statistically significant, they may not be *practically significant*. Here is one area where statistics is a bit of an art form and a science.

Practical significance expresses the meaningfulness or importance of differences in statistical analysis. While statistical significance indicates whether an effect is likely due to chance, practical significance assesses whether the effect has any meaningful impact in a practical context.

Calculating practical significance often involves considering the *effect size*, which quantifies the magnitude of the observed difference or relationship. When testing with large samples, it is worth considering including a measure of effect size and statistical significance. There are various methods to measure effect size. Cohen's *d* is a commonly employed method that takes the following form.

$$d = \frac{\bar{x}_1 - \bar{x}_2}{s_p}$$

$$s_p = \sqrt{\frac{(n_1 - 1) \times s_1^2 + (n_2 - 1) \times s_2^2}{n_1 + n_2 - 2}}$$

where *d* is Cohen's d, which is calculated as the difference between two group means divided by pooled standard deviation s_p. Given its relative nature, it is suggested that Cohen's *d* is described with loose terminology. There are several recommendations in the literature to describe Cohen's *d*. One option is to report a difference of around 0.2 as "small" indicating a relatively small difference or effect, 0.05 as "medium" indicating a moderate effect, and 0.8 or higher as "large" indicating a substantial effect.

Perhaps we're measuring the cognitive function scores of a group of nursing home patients before and after a series of cognitive exercises. We might be interested in the magnitude of the difference, measured through practical and statistical significance. An implementation of Cohen's d in Python and R using this representative example is as follows:

Python

```
import numpy as np

before_training = np.array([25, 28, 22, 23, 26, 27, 20,
24, 21, 29])
after_training = np.array([30, 32, 26, 28, 31, 33, 25,
29, 27, 34])

mean_before = np.mean(before_training)
mean_after = np.mean(after_training)
std_before = np.std(before_training, ddof=1)  # ddof=1
for sample standard deviation
std_after = np.std(after_training, ddof=1)
```

```
pooled_std = np.sqrt((((len(before_training)-1) * std_
before**2 + (len(after_training)-1) * std_after**2) /
(len(before_training) + len(after_training) - 2))
cohens_d = (mean_after - mean_before) / pooled_std
print("Cohen's d: {:.2f}".format(cohens_d))
```

R

We can use the effsize package in R for a simplified implementation.

```
library(effsize)

before_training <- c(25, 28, 22, 23, 26, 27, 20, 24, 21,
29)
after_training <- c(30, 32, 26, 28, 31, 33, 25, 29, 27,
34)

cohen_result <- cohen.d(before_training, after_training,
pooled = TRUE)

print(cohen_result)
```

Odds ratios, risk differences, and risk ratios are other examples of effect size measures, which we will discuss in more detail in the Chapter 7.

For now, it is important to remember that practical significance can vary depending on the situation. An effect considered practically significant in one context might not be in another. Balancing statistical significance and practical significance helps ensure that research findings have real-world relevance and are not just statistically detectable but also meaningful and actionable.

Corrections for Multiple Tests

It is not uncommon to conduct multiple tests on a variable of interest. However, we must be cautious in these scenarios, as more tests increase the likelihood of finding a spurious relationship in the data—that is, the chances of obtaining a Type I error rise considerably.

Let's consider a situation in which an analyst evaluates the effectiveness of a medical intervention on various process measures using the PQRS (Physician Quality Reporting System) measure set, which is used within the MIPS program.

The analyst is evaluating the potential impact of an educational intervention on physicians' adherence to three different process measures, evaluating adherence to 1) blood pressure screening guidelines, 2) influenza vaccination recommendations, and 3) tobacco cessation counseling guidelines.

He decides to conduct separate hypothesis tests to determine whether the intervention significantly affects each process measure's adherence rate. For each test, he sets a conventional significance level of $\alpha = 0.05$; however, if these tests are performed without any correction, the cumulative chance of making at least one Type I error across all three tests increases, leading to a larger *familywise error rate* (FWER). The familywise error rate refers to the probability of making at least one Type I error in a set of multiple hypothesis tests—incorrectly rejecting our null hypothesis in favor of the alternate hypothesis. When conducting multiple hypothesis tests simultaneously, there's an increased chance of observing at least one significant result by random chance, even if all null hypotheses are true. The familywise error rate controls this overall error rate to maintain the overall significance level of the tests. With three tests, the uncorrected familywise error rate is $1 - (1 - \alpha)^3$, or .143, which is greater than the desired overall significance level of 0.05. This means there is a higher chance of making a false discovery across all tests.

The most common approach to controlling the familywise error rate is to apply a correction method to the individual *p*-values obtained from the individual tests. The Bonferroni correction can be used to control for the familywise error rate. For each test, the desired overall significance level ($\alpha = 0.05$) is divided by the number of tests (three in this case), resulting in a corrected significance level of $\alpha_{Bonferroni} == 0.05 / 3 = 0.0167$.

Using the Bonferroni correction lowers the chance of making a Type I error across all tests while maintaining a more stringent threshold for each test. This helps ensure that the overall familywise error rate remains below the desired level and that the evaluation of the process measures is more reliable. More robust correction methods, such as the Holm-Bonferroni method, can also be considered (a correction that does not make the assumption that all variables are independent).

Considering Case Mix

We have been evaluating the crude mean or proportion of patient events in many of the examples above. If we assume that the patient mix (i.e., the clinical and demographic distributions of the patient population) between the two evaluated values are the same, then such tests can be useful. In many cases, however, we cannot assume that the populations are comparable. An entire chapter on "Risk Standardization" is dedicated to this subject later in this book. For now, it is important to be aware of the concept of patient mix and the dangers of misleading or incorrect conclusions that can occur if the populations being compared are materially different.

TABLE 3.5

One-Sample z-Test for Means

Assumptions:
- The population standard deviation σ is known
- The population distribution is approximately normal or the number of samples is $n \geq 30$

Set Up Hypothesis	Python Implementation	R Implementation

Null Hypothesis (H_0): $\mu = \mu_0$
 	
 Alternate Hypothesis (H_a):
 Left Tail: $\mu < \mu_0$
 Right Tail: $\mu > \mu_0$
 Two Tail: $\mu \neq \mu_0$
 	
 Set the Significance Level
 $\alpha = .05$
 	
 Calculate Test Statistic
 $z = \dfrac{\bar{x} - \mu_0}{\dfrac{\sigma}{\sqrt{n}}}$
 	
 Calculate the p-value
 Left Tail: $p = P(Z \leq z)$
 Right Left:
 $p = P(Z \geq z)$
 Two Tail:
 $p = 2 \times P(Z \geq \lvert z \rvert)$
 	
 Make a decision
 Reject Null if $p < \alpha$
	<pre>import numpy as np
	from scipy.stats import norm
	data = np.array([10.2, 9.8, 10.4, 10.0,
	10.1, 10.3, 9.9])
	hypothesized_mean = 10.0
	sample_mean = np.mean(data)
	sample_std = np.std(data, ddof=1)
	#Set Significance Level
	alpha = .05
	#Calculate Test Statistic
	test_statistic = (sample_mean -
	hypothesized_mean) / (sample_std /
	np.sqrt(len(data)))
	#Calculate p-Value
	#Left Tail:
	p_value = norm.cdf(test_statistic)
	#Right Tail
	p_value = 1 - norm.cdf(test_statistic)
	#Two Tail:
	p_value = 2 * (1 - norm.
	cdf(abs(test_statistic)))
	Make a Decision
	if p_value < alpha:
	    print("Reject the null hypothesis.")
	else:
	    print("Fail to reject the null
	hypothesis.")</pre>
		<pre>data <- c(10.2, 9.8, 10.4, 10.0, 10.1, 10.3,
		9.9)
		hypothesized_mean <- 10.0
		sample_mean <- mean(data)
		sample_std <- sd(data)
		sample_size <- length(data)
		# Set significance level
		alpha <- 0.05
		# Calculate the test statistic
		test_statistic <- (sample_mean -
		hypothesized_mean) / (sample_std /
		sqrt(sample_size))
		#Calculate p-Value
		#Left Tail:
		p_value <- pnorm(test_statistic)
		#Right Tail
		# Calculate p-value for the right tail
		p_value <- 1 - pnorm(test_statistic)
		#Two Tail:
		p_value <- 2 * (1
		- pnorm(abs(test_statistic)))
		# Make a decision
		if (p_value < alpha) {
		    print("Reject the null hypothesis.")
		} else {
		    print("Fail to reject the null
		hypothesis.")}</pre>

TABLE 3.6

One-Sample t-Test for Means

Assumptions:
- The population standard deviation σ is unknown.
- The sample distribution is approximately normal or the number of samples is $n < 30$.

Set Up Hypothesis	Python Implementation	R Implementation

Null Hypothesis (H_0): $\mu = \mu_0$
 	
 Alternate Hypothesis (H_0):
 Left Tail: $\mu < \mu_0$
 Right Tail: $\mu > \mu_0$
 Two Tail: $\mu \neq \mu_0$
 	
 Set the Significance Level
 $\alpha = .05$
 	
 Calculate Test Statistic
 $t = \dfrac{\bar{x} - \mu_0}{\frac{s}{\sqrt{n}}}$
 	
 Calculate the p-value
 Left Tail: $p = P(T \leq t)$
 Right Tail: $p = P(T \geq t)$
 Two Tail: $p = 2 \times P(T \geq \lvert t \rvert)$
 	
 Make a decision
 Reject H_0 if $p < \alpha$
	<pre>import numpy as np
	from scipy.stats import ttest_1samp
	data = np.array([10.2, 9.8, 10.4,
	10.0, 10.1, 10.3, 9.91)
	hypothesized_mean = 10.0
	#Set significance level
	alpha = .05
	#Calcualte test statistic
	#Left Tail:
	t_statistic, p_value =
	ttest_1samp(data, hypothesized_mean,
	alternative='less')
	#Right Tail:
	t_statistic, p_value =
	ttest_1samp(data, hypothesized_mean,
	alternative='greater')
	#Two Tail:
	t_statistic, p_value =
	ttest_1samp(data, hypothesized_mean,
	alternative='two-sided')
	#Make a decision
	if p_value < alpha:
	    print("Reject the null hypothesis.")
	else:
	    print("Fail to reject the null
	    hypothesis.")</pre>
		<pre>data <- c(10.2, 9.8, 10.4, 10.0, 10.1, 10.3,
		9.9)
		hypothesized_mean <- 10.0
		# Set significance level
		alpha <- 0.05
		# Perform one-sample t-tests
		# Left Tail
		test_left <- t.test(data, mu = hypothesized_
		mean, alternative = "less")
		# Right Tail
		test_right <- t.test(data, mu = hypothesized_
		mean, alternative = "greater")
		# Two-Tail
		test_two_tail <- t.test(data, mu =
		hypothesized_mean, alternative = "two.sided")
		# Access the p_value
		p_value <- test_left$p.value
		p_value <- test_right$p.value
		p_value <- test_two_tail$p.value
		#Make a decision
		if (p_value < alpha) {
		    print("Reject the null hypothesis.")
		} else {
		    print("Fail to reject the null hypothesis..")
		}</pre>

TABLE 3.7

Two-sample t-test for Means (Pooled Variance)

Assumptions:

- The standard deviation for σ_1 and σ_2 is unknown.
- The samples are independent.
- The sample distributions for the two samples are approximately normal.
- The variance across the two samples is equal.

Set Up Hypothesis	Python Implementation	R Implementation
| *Null Hypothesis* $(H_0): \mu_1 - \mu_2 = 0$<br><br>*Alternate Hypothesis* $(H_a)$:<br><br>Left Tail: $\mu_1 - \mu_2 < 0$<br><br>Right Tail: $\mu_1 - \mu_2 > 0$<br><br>Two Tail: $\mu_1 - \mu_2 = 0$<br><br>**Set the Significance Level**<br>$\alpha = .05$<br><br>**Calculate Test Statistic**<br>$$s_p = \sqrt{\dfrac{(n_1-1)s_1^2 + (n_2-1)s_2^2}{n_1 + n_2 - 2}}$$<br><br>$$t = \dfrac{\bar{x}_1 - \bar{x}_2 - 0}{s_p\sqrt{\dfrac{1}{n_1} + \dfrac{1}{n_2}}}$$<br><br>**Calculate the *p*-value**<br><br>Left Tail: $p = P(T \leq t)$<br><br>Right Tail: $p = P(T \geq t)$<br><br>Two Tail: $p = 2 \times P(T \geq \lvert t \rvert)$<br><br>**Make a decision**<br>Reject $H_0$ if $p < \alpha$ | ```python
import numpy as np
from scipy.stats import ttest_ind
group1 = np.array([23, 27, 30, 25, 28])
group2 = np.array([18, 20, 22, 17, 21])
#Set the significance level
alpha = 0.05
# Left Tail
t_statistic, p_value =
ttest_ind(group1, group2,
alternative='less',equal_var=True)
# Right Tail
t_statistic, p_value =
ttest_ind(group1, group2,
alternative='greater',equal_var=True)
# Two Tail
t_statistic, p_value =
ttest_ind(group1, group2,
alternative='two-sided',equal_var=True)
# Make a Decision
if p_value < alpha:
    print("Reject the null hypothesis.")
else:
    print("Fail to reject the null
hypothesis.")
``` | ```r
# Data setup
group1 <- c(23, 27, 30, 25, 28)
group2 <- c(18, 20, 22, 17, 21)
# Set significance level
alpha <- 0.05
# Perform two-sample t-tests
# Left Tail
test_left <- t.test(group1, group2,
alternative = "less", var.equal = TRUE)
# Right Tail
test_right <- t.test(group1, group2,
alternative = "greater", var.equal = TRUE)
# Two-Tail
test_two_tail <- t.test(group1, group2,
alternative = "two.sided", var.equal = TRUE)
#Access the p value
p_value <- test_left$p.value
p_value <- test_right$p.value
p_value <- test_two_tail$p.value
# Make a decision
if (p_value < alpha) {
    print("Reject the null hypothesis.")
} else {
    print("Fail to reject the null
hypothesis.")
}
``` |

TABLE 3.8

Two-sample t-test for Means (Unpooled Variance)

Assumptions:
- The standard deviation for σ_1 and σ_2 is unknown.
- The samples are independent (each observation in one group should not be influenced by or dependent on observations in the other group).
- The sample distributions for the two samples are approximately normal.
- The variance across the two samples is not equal.

Set Up Hypothesis	Python Implementation	R Implementation

Null Hypothesis (H_0):
 $\mu_1 - \mu_2 = 0$
 Alternate Hypothesis (H_a):
 Left Tail: $\mu_1 - \mu_2 < 0$
 Right Tail: $\mu_1 - \mu_2 > 0$
 Two Tail: $\mu_1 - \mu_2 = 0$
 Set the Significance Level
 $\alpha = .05$
 Calculate Test Statistic
 $t = \dfrac{\bar{x}_1 - \bar{x}_2 - 0}{\sqrt{\dfrac{s_1^2}{n_1} + \dfrac{s_2^2}{n_2}}}$
 	
 Calculate the *p*-value
 Left Tail: $p = P(T \leq t)$
 Right Tail: $p = P(T \geq t)$
 Two Tail: $p = 2 \times P(T \geq \|t\|)$
 	
 Make a decision
 Reject H_0 if $p < \alpha$
	```python```
	`import numpy as np`
	`from scipy.stats import ttest_ind`
	`group1 = np.array([23, 27, 30, 25, 28])`
	`group2 = np.array([18, 20, 22, 17, 21])`
	`# Set the significance level`
	`alpha = 0.05`
	`# Left Tail`
	`t_statistic, p_value =`
	`ttest_ind(group1, group2,`
	`alternative='less', equal_var=False)`
	`# Right Tail`
	`t_statistic, p_value =`
	`ttest_ind(group1, group2,`
	`alternative='greater', equal_var=False)`
	`# Two Tail`
	`t_statistic, p_value =`
	`ttest_ind(group1, group2,`
	`alternative='two-sided',equal_var=False)`
	`# Make a decision`
	`if p_value < alpha:`
	`    print("Reject the null hypothesis.")`
	`else:`
	`    print("Fail to reject the null`
	`hypothesis.")`
		`# Data setup`
		`group1 <- c(23, 27, 30, 25, 28)`
		`group2 <- c(18, 20, 22, 17, 21)`
		`# Set significance level`
		`alpha <- 0.05`
		`# Perform independent two-sample t-tests`
		`# Left Tail`
		`test_left <- t.test(group1, group2,`
		`alternative = "less", var.equal = FALSE)`
		`# Right Tail`
		`test_right <- t.test(group1, group2,`
		`alternative = "greater", var.equal = FALSE)`
		`# Two-Tail`
		`test_two_tail <- t.test(group1, group2,`
		`alternative = "two.sided", var.equal = FALSE)`
		`# Access p-values`
		`p_value <- test_left$p.value`
		`p_value <- test_right$p.value`
		`p_value <- test_two_tail$p.value`
		`# Make a decision`
		`if (p_value < alpha) {`
		`    print("Reject the null hypothesis.")`
		`} else {`
		`    print("Fail to reject the null`
		`hypothesis.")`
		`}`

TABLE 3.9

Paired Difference t-test for Means

Assumptions:
- The distribution of the differences is approximately equal
- The number of pairs is ≥30

Set Up Hypothesis	Python Implementation	R Implementation
| *Null Hypothesis* $(H_0)$: <br> $\mu_d = 0$ <br> *Alternate* <br> *Hypothesis* $(H_a)$: <br> Left Tail: $\mu_d < 0$ <br> Right Tail: $\mu_d > 0$ <br> Two Tail: $\mu_d \neq 0$ <br> **Set the Significance** <br> **Level** <br> $\alpha = .05$ <br> **Calculate Test** <br> **Statistic** <br> $t = \dfrac{\bar{d} - 0}{\dfrac{s}{\sqrt{n}}}$ <br><br> **Calculate the p-value** <br> Left Tail: $p = P(T \leq t)$ <br> Right Tail: <br> $p = P(T \geq t)$ <br> Two Tail: <br> $p = 2 \times P(T \geq \|t\|)$ <br> **Make a Decision** <br> Reject $H_0$ if $p < \alpha$ | ```
import numpy as np
    from scipy.stats import ttest_rel
    # Data for paired samples
before = np.array([12.2, 11.8, 10.4,
11.0, 10.5])
after = np.array([11.0, 11.5, 9.8,
10.0, 9.5])
#Set significance level
alpha = 0.05
    # Calculate test statistic and p-value
    # Left tail
t_statistic, p_value = ttest_
rel(before, after, alternative='less')
    # Right tail
t_statistic, p_value =
ttest_rel(before, after,
alternative='greater')
    # Two tail
t_statistic, p_value =
ttest_rel(before, after,
alternative='two-sided')
    # Make a decision
    if p_value < alpha:
        print("Reject the null hypothesis in
favor of the alternate hypothesis.")
    else:
        print("Fail to reject the null
hypothesis.")
``` | ```
before <- c(12.2, 11.8, 10.4, 11.0, 10.5)
after <- c(11.0, 11.5, 9.8, 10.0, 9.5)
# Set significance level
alpha <- 0.05
# Perform paired t-tests
# Left Tail
test_left <- t.test(before, after,
paired = TRUE, alternative = "less")
# Right Tail
test_right <- t.test(before, after,
paired = TRUE, alternative =
"greater")
# Two-Tail
test_two_tail <- t.test(before, after,
paired = TRUE, alternative = "two.
sided")
# Access p-values
p_value <- test_left$p.value
p_value <- test_right$p.value
p_value <- test_two_tail$p.value
# Make a decision
if (p_value < alpha) {
    print("Reject the null hypothesis.")
} else {
    print("Fail to reject the null
hypothesis.")
}
``` |

TABLE 3.10

One-Sample z-Test for Proportions

Assumptions:
- Have at least five successes and non-successes: $np_0 \geq 10$ and $n(1-p_0) \geq 10$

Set Up Hypothesis	Python Implementation	R Implementation

Null Hypothesis (H_0): $\mu = \mu_0$
 	
 Alternate Hypothesis (H_a):
 Left Tail: $\mu < \mu_0$
 Right Tail: $\mu > \mu_0$
 Two Tail: $\mu \neq \mu_0$
 	
 Set the Significance Level
 $\alpha = .05$
 	
 Calculate Test Statistic
 	
 $z = \dfrac{\hat{p} - p_0}{\sqrt{\dfrac{p_0(1-p_0)}{n}}}$
 	
 Calculate the p-value
 	
 Left Tail:
 $p = P(Z \leq z)$
 	
 Right Tail:
 $p = P(Z \geq z)$
 	
 Two Tail:
 $p = 2 \times P(Z \geq \lvert z \rvert)$
 	
 Make a decision
 Reject H_0 if $p < \alpha$
	<pre>import numpy as np
	from statsmodels.stats.proportion import
	proportions_ztest
	successes_sample = 25
	sample_size = 100
	null_hypothesis_proportion = 0.5
	# Set the significance level
	alpha = 0.05
	# Calculate test statistic and p-value
	#Left Tail
	z_statistic, p_value = proportions_
	ztest(successes_sample, sample_
	size, null_hypothesis_proportion,
	alternative='smaller')
	# Right Tail
	z_statistic, p_value = proportions_
	ztest(successes_sample, sample_
	size, null_hypothesis_proportion,
	alternative='larger')
	# Two-tail
	z_statistic, p_value = proportions_
	ztest(successes_sample, sample_size,
	null_hypothesis_proportion)
	# Make a decision
	if p_value < alpha:
	    print("Reject the null hypothesis in
	favor of the alternate hypothesis.")
	else:
	    print("Fail to reject the null
	hypothesis.")</pre>
		<pre>successes_sample <- 25
		sample_size <- 100
		null_hypothesis_proportion <- 0.5
		# Set the significance level
		alpha = 0.05
		# Calculate test statistic
		test_two_tail <- prop.test(successes_sample,
		sample_size, p = null_hypothesis_proportion,
		alternative = "two.sided", correct = FALSE)
		# Left Tail
		test_left <- prop.test(successes_sample,
		sample_size, p = null_hypothesis_proportion,
		alternative = "less", correct = FALSE)
		# Right Tail
		test_right <- prop.test(successes_sample,
		sample_size, p = null_hypothesis_proportion,
		alternative = "greater", correct = FALSE)
		# Extract p-values
		p_value <- test_two_tail$p.value
		p_value <- test_left$p.value
		p_value <- test_right$p.value
		# Make a decision
		if (p_value < alpha) {
		    print("Reject the null hypothesis.")
		} else {
		    print("Fail to reject the null hypothesis.")
		}</pre>

TABLE 3.11

Two-Sample z-test for Proportions

Assumptions:

- Have at least ten successes and non-successes in each sample: $n_1 p_1, n_1(1-p_1), n_2 p_2, n_2(1-p_2) \geq 10$

Set Up Hypothesis	Python Implementation	R Implementation
Hypothesis (H_0): $p_1 = p_2$	`import numpy as np`	`successes_sample1 <- 45`
	`from statsmodels.stats.proportion import`	`sample_size1 <- 150`
Alternate Hypothesis (H_a):	`proportions_ztest`	`successes_sample2 <- 30`
Left Tail: $p_1 < p_2$	`successes_sample1 = 45`	`sample_size2 <- 120`
Right Tail: $p_1 > p_2$	`sample_size1 = 150`	`successes <- c(successes_sample1,`
Two Tail: $p_1 \neq p_2$	`successes_sample2 = 30`	`successes_sample2)`
Set the Significance Level	`sample_size2 = 120`	`sample_sizes <- c(sample_size1,`
$\alpha = .05$	`successes = np.array([successes_sample1,`	`sample_size2)`
Calculate Test Statistic	`successes_sample2])`	`# Set significance level`
	`sample_sizes = np.array([sample_size1,`	`alpha <- 0.05`
	`sample_size2])`	`# Left Tail Test`
$z = \dfrac{\hat{p}_1 - \hat{p}_2 - 0}{\sqrt{\hat{p}(1-\hat{p})\left(\dfrac{1}{n_1} + \dfrac{1}{n_2}\right)}}$	`#Set the significance level`	`test_left <- prop.test(successes,`
	`alpha = 0.05`	`sample_sizes, alternative = "less",`
	`# Calculate Test Statistic`	`correct = FALSE)`
	`# Left tail`	`# Right Tail Test`
$\hat{p} = \dfrac{x_1 + x_2}{n_1 + n_2}$	`z_statistic, p_value = proportions_`	`test_right <- prop.test(successes,`
Calculate the p-value	`ztest(successes, sample_sizes,`	`sample_sizes, alternative = "greater",`
Left Tail: $p = P(Z \leq z)$	`alternative='less')`	`correct = FALSE)`
	`# Right tail`	`# Two-Tailed Test`
Right Tail: $p = P(Z \geq z)$	`z_statistic, p_value = proportions_`	`test_two_tail <- prop.test(successes,`
	`ztest(successes, sample_sizes,`	`sample_sizes, alternative = "two.`
Two Tail: $p = 2 \times P(Z \geq |z|)$	`alternative='greater')`	`sided", correct = FALSE)`
	`# Two tail`	
Make a Decision	`z_statistic, p_value = proportions_`	
Reject H_0 if $p < \alpha$	`ztest(successes, sample_sizes,`	
	`alternative='two-sided')`	

(Continued)

TABLE 3.11 (CONTINUED)

Set Up Hypothesis	Python Implementation	R Implementation
| | ```
# Make a decision
if p_value < alpha:
    print("Reject the null hypothesis in
favor of the alternate hypothesis.")
else:
    print("Fail to reject the null
hypothesis.")
``` | ```
# Extract the p-value
p_value<- test_left$p.value
p_value <- test_right$p.value
p_value <- test_two_tail$p.value
# Decision for each test
if (p_value < alpha) {
    cat("Reject the null
hypothesis.")
} else {
    cat("Fail to reject the null
hypothesis.")
}
``` |

Additional Resources

Casella, G., & Berger, R. L. (2024). *Statistical Inference* (2nd ed.). Chapman & Hall/CRC Texts in Statistical Science.
Wasserman, L. (2010). *All of Statistics: A Concise Course in Statistical Inference* (Springer Texts in Statistics). Springer.

4

Confidence Intervals

Sample means and proportions inherently have some degree of error. As mentioned in the previous Chapter, if we repeatedly sample the length of stay for 30 med/surg patients, the mean of each sample can vary considerably. This variation across samples is a result of error in the sample itself and does not reflect any true difference in overall length of stay. While we cannot know the true population length of stay in many cases, we can estimate the range of values with some degree of confidence in which the population mean would exist (accounting for the potential error that we would expect from the sample). In the context of our length of stay example, an upper and lower 95% confidence interval would provide a range of length of stay values in which the true population mean would exist. We can state that we are 95% confident that the true length of stay is within the upper and lower confidence limits.

A confidence interval is calculated by padding the sample statistic (e.g., a sample mean or proportion) with a margin of error. for example, the confidence interval of a sample mean can be expressed as follows:

$$\bar{x} \pm \text{margin of error}$$

While a proportion might be expressed as

$$\hat{p} \pm \text{margin of error}$$

Furthermore, the margin of error itself is formed from two components—a multiplier and standard error:

$$\text{margin of error} = \text{multipler} \times \text{standarderror}$$

The multiplier and the standard error are combined to form the overall margin of error. Let's look at the confidence interval for a sample mean (such as length of stay) as an example.

DOI: 10.1201/9781003609759-4

Sample   Standard
Statistic   Error

Multiplier

$$\bar{x} \pm z_{a/2} \times \frac{\sigma}{\sqrt{n}}$$

Margin of Error

Here $\bar{x}$ is the sample statistic (or sample mean). The margin of error $z_{a/2} \times \frac{\sigma}{\sqrt{n}}$ is comprised of the multiplier $z_{a/2}$ and standard error $\frac{\sigma}{\sqrt{n}}$. Recall that if we take repeated samples and calculate the means of each of those samples, the standard deviation of those means approximates the standard error.

A rule about standard deviations (or standard errors when evaluating means) is that 95% of the sample means will be within approximately two (closer to 1.96 to be more precise) standard deviations from the true mean. Let's look at the below figure to help us untangle this mess (Figure 4.1).

Here, we show five samples each comprised of 30 med/surg patients. For each of the 30 patients, we calculate a mean and standard deviation (as indicated by the dot and whiskers below the curve). If we repeated these samples 100 times, roughly 95% of the sample means would be within two standard deviations (or standard errors) of the true mean (indicated by the $z = 1.96$ boundaries on the curve). The multiplier indicates the number of standard deviations from the mean we set based on our desired confidence level.

When deciding on the multiplier, a helpful estimate is to use the 68-95-99.7 rule, which states that approximately 68% of the data will be within one standard deviation and 95% will be within two standard deviations. If we want to be 99.7% confident that the true mean is within our confidence intervals, our multiplier would be increased to a value closer to 3.

Of course, these are rough estimates of multipliers, and we can use software (or tables) to identify a more precise multiplier.

Below is an example of computing a z-score of 1.96 (approximately 2) with a 95% confidence level in Python

```
import scipy.stats as st
confidence_level = .95
z_score = st.norm.ppf(1 - (1 - confidence_level) / 2)
```

The `stats.norm.ppf` function is the probability mass function for a normal distribution. The probability mass function gives us the z-score that marks the point in the distribution where 95% of the data is represented. This intuitively seems correct, but it is not! We are interested in the margin of error

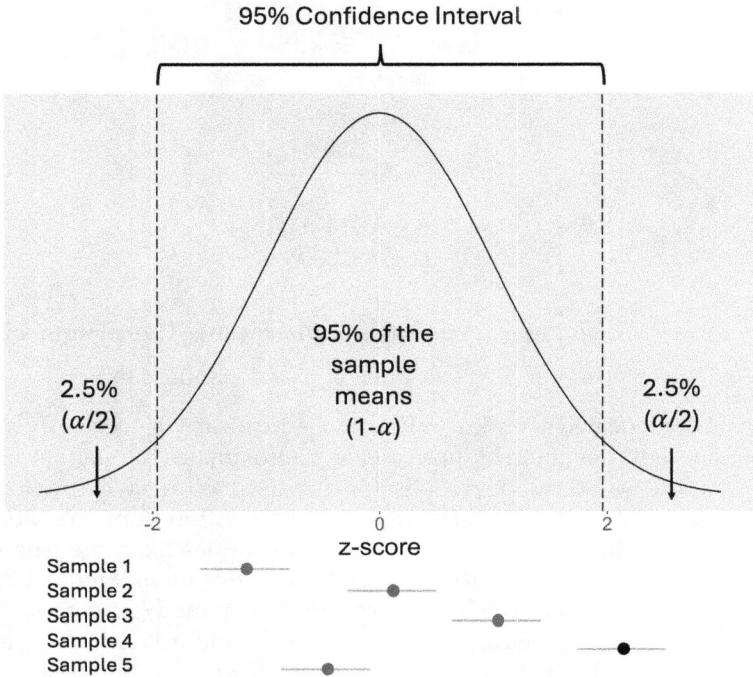

FIGURE 4.1
An example of a 95% confidence interval using a normal distribution.

on both sides (recall that we add and subtract the margin of error to determine the confidence interval), and therefore, we must split the 5% to both tails. Said another way, we want to identify the 97.5% of data on each side of the distribution to obtain a left and right confidence interval computed by $1 - (1 - \text{confidence level})/2$. We will also see the z value represented in notation as $z_{a/2}$ which denotes the splitting of alpha (e.g., .05) to each side.

Equivalently in R, we can use the qnorm function analogous to stats. norm.ppf in Python to calculate the cumulative probability (assuming an normal distribution):

```
confidence_level <- 0.95
z_score <- qnorm(1 - (1 - confidence_level) / 2)
```

Let's walk through a representative example using proportion data. A family practice physician has implemented some operational changes to ensure that diabetic patients receive kidney health evaluation during their office visits (a MIPS-eligible measure). Upon implementing the new policy, the physician begins evaluating measure compliance—that is, the proportion of diabetic patients receiving kidney health evaluations. The sample size is small, and she knows there will be some degree of error in the sample proportion. She

TABLE 4.1

Demonstration of Narrowing Confidence Intervals with Increased Sample Size

Week	Sample Proportion	Lower 95% CI	Upper 95% CI	Number of Kidney Health Evaluations	Number of Diabetic Patients Seen
1	0.778	.506	0.999	7	9
2	0.81	0.642	0.977	17	21
3	0.829	0.704	0.953	29	35
4	0.824	0.719	0.928	42	51
5	0.83	0.751	0.920	61	73
52	0.83	0.803	0.856	647	780

conducts a confidence interval the week after the policy change and each week thereafter to understand the error range in the observed proportion. In the first week, the physician saw nine diabetic patients and, of those patients, conducted seven kidney health evaluations.

As shown in Table 4.1, the error range (or confidence interval) in the first week is quite large, with a confidence interval ranging from .506 to .999. Given the range of error with this estimate, she reserves judgment. With each week, the cumulative number of people with diabetes seen increases until week five, where she has evaluated 61 out of 73 diabetic patients. By this point, the confidence interval has narrowed considerably, ranging from .751 to .920 for a sample mean of .83. As the sample size increases (i.e., more diabetic patients are seen), the degree of error in our estimate will narrow.

A year passes, and measure compliance is reassessed. Having conducted 647 evaluations out of 780 diabetic patients, she reports to her peers that measure compliance for kidney health evaluation for the year is 83%. She qualifies this statistic with "95% CI [80.3–85.6]", indicating the confidence level (95%) and the confidence interval (CI) [80.3–85.6].

Her code is as follows:

```
import statsmodels.api as sm
from statsmodels.stats.proportion import proportion_
confint
proportion_confint(count=647, nobs=780, alpha=0.05)
```

which we can also write in R:

```
result <- prop.test(x = 647, n = 780, conf.level = 0.95)
result$conf.int
```

As with hypothesis tests, we must choose the most appropriate formula for the parameter we are attempting to estimate through the confidence interval. Table 4.2 can serve as a guide for the most common confidence interval scenarios. These tables contain the assumptions for each test, the formulas, and an example implementation using Python and R.

TABLE 4.2

Confidence Interval Methods with Implementations in Python and R

CI Type	Python Implementation	R Implementation

Estimated Parameter: Population mean μ
 Sample Statistic: Sample mean $\bar{x}$
 Confidence Interval Formula:
 $\bar{x} \pm z_{\alpha/2} \times \dfrac{\sigma}{\sqrt{n}}$
 	
 Assumptions:
 The population standard deviation σ is known
 	
 The population distribution is approximately normal or the number of samples is $n \geq 30$
	<pre>import numpy as np
	import scipy.stats as st
	# Sample data
	data = np.array([23, 27, 19, 31, 25, 29,
	22, 18, 24, 28])
	# Known population standard deviation
	known_std_dev = 4.5
	# Set confidence level
	confidence_level = 0.95
	# Calculate sample mean
	sample_mean = np.mean(data)
	# Calculate the standard error
	standard_error = known_std_dev /
	np.sqrt(len(data))
	# Calculate the margin of error
	z_score = st.norm.ppf(1 - (1 - confidence_
	level) / 2)
	margin_of_error = z_score * standard_error
	# Calculate the confidence interval
	lower_bound = sample_mean - margin_of_error
	upper_bound = sample_mean + margin_of_error
	print("Margin of Error:", margin_of_error)
	print(f"Confidence Interval: ({lower_
	bound:.3f}, {upper_bound:.3f})")</pre>
		<pre># Sample data
		data <- c(23, 27, 19, 31, 25, 29, 22, 18,
		24, 28)
		# Known population standard deviation
		known_std_dev <- 4.5
		# Set confidence level
		confidence_level <- 0.95
		# Calculate sample mean
		sample_mean <- mean(data)
		# Calculate the standard error
		standard_error <- known_std_dev /
		sqrt(length(data))
		# Calculate the z-score for the given
		confidence level
		z_score <- qnorm(1 - (1 - confidence_level)
		/ 2)
		# Calculate the margin of error
		margin_of_error <- z_score * standard_error
		# Calculate the confidence interval
		lower_bound <- sample_mean -
		margin_of_error
		upper_bound <- sample_mean +
		margin_of_error
		cat("Margin of Error:", margin_of_error,
		"\n")
		cat(sprintf("95%% Confidence Interval:
		(%.3f, %.3f)\n", lower_bound, upper_bound))</pre>

| Estimated Parameter: Population mean μ<br>Sample Statistic: *Sample mean* $\bar{x}$<br>Confidence Interval Formula:<br><br>$$\bar{x} \pm t_{\alpha/2, n-1} \times \frac{s}{\sqrt{n}}$$<br><br>Assumptions:<br>The population standard deviation σ is known<br>The population distribution is approximately normal or the number of samples is n ≥ 30 | ```python
import numpy as np
from scipy import stats
# Sample data
data = np.array([22, 25, 28, 30, 32, 35,
38, 40, 42, 45])
# Calculate sample mean, standard error,
and degrees of freedom
sample_mean = np.mean(data)
standard_error = stats.sem(data)
degrees_freedom = len(data) - 1
# Calculate the 95% confidence interval
confidence_level = 0.95
confidence_interval =
stats.t.interval(confidence_level,
df=degrees_freedom, loc=sample_mean,
scale=standard_error)
# Print results
print("Sample Mean (x̄):", sample_mean)
print("t-Statistic:", stats.t.ppf((1 +
confidence_level) / 2, df=degrees_freedom))
print("95% Confidence Interval:",
confidence_interval)
``` | ```r
# Sample data for two groups
group_1 <- c(22, 25, 28, 30, 32)
group_2 <- c(38, 40, 42, 45, 48)
# Perform a two-sample t-test to get the
confidence interval for the difference
between means
t_test_result <- t.test(group_1, group_2,
var.equal = FALSE, conf.level = 0.95)
# Print the results
cat("t-Score:", t_test_result$statistic,
"\n")
cat("Degrees of Freedom:", t_test_
result$parameter, "\n")
cat("Margin of Error:", (t_test_
result$conf.int[2] - t_test_
result$estimate), "\n")

cat("95% Confidence Interval: (", t_
test_result$conf.int[1], ", ", t_test_
result$conf.int[2], ")\n", sep = "")
``` |
| Estimated Parameter: Difference in population means μ₁ - μ₂ | ```python
import numpy as np
from scipy import stats
# Sample data for two groups
group_1 = np.array([22, 25, 28, 30, 32])
group_2 = np.array([38, 40, 42, 45, 48])
# Calculate sample means and standard
deviations
``` | |

(Continued)
```

TABLE 4.2 (CONTINUED)

CI Type	Python Implementation	R Implementation

Sample Statistic: Difference in sample means $\bar{x}_1 - \bar{x}_2$	`std_dev_1 = np.std(group_1, ddof=1)`
	`std_dev_2 = np.std(group_2, ddof=1)`
	`# Calculate degrees of freedom for unpooled variance t-test`
	`degrees_freedom_1 = len(group_1) - 1`
	`degrees_freedom_2 = len(group_2) - 1`
		`# Sample data for two groups`
		`group_1 <- c(22, 25, 28, 30, 32)`
		`group_2 <- c(38, 40, 42, 45, 48)`
		`# Perform a two-sample t-test for unequal variances (Welch's t-test)`
		`t_test_result <- t.test(group_1, group_2, var.equal = FALSE, conf.level = 0.95)`

Confidence Interval Formula: $\bar{x}_1 - \bar{x}_2 \pm t_{\alpha/2} \times \sqrt{\dfrac{s_1^2}{n_1} + \dfrac{s_2^2}{n_2}}$	`# Calculate t-score for a 95% confidence interval`
	`confidence_level = 0.95`
	`t_score = stats.t.ppf((1 + confidence_level) / 2, df=min(degrees_freedom_1, degrees_freedom_2))`
		`# Extract the relevant values`
		`t_statistic <- t_test_result$statistic`
		`degrees_freedom <- t_test_result$parameter`
		`conf_int <- t_test_result$conf.int`
		`mean_difference <- t_test_result$estimate[1] - t_test_result$estimate[2]`

Assumptions:
The standard deviation for σ_1 and σ_2 is unknown
The samples are independent
The sample distributions for the two samples are approximately normal
The variance across the two samples is not equal
	`# Calculate standard error of the difference between means`
	`standard_error_diff = np.sqrt((std_dev_1**2 / len(group_1)) + (std_dev_2**2 / len(group_2)))`
	`# Calculate margin of error`
	`margin_of_error = t_score * standard_error_diff`
	`# Calculate confidence interval`
	`mean_difference = mean_1 - mean_2`
	`confidence_interval_lower = mean_difference - margin_of_error`
	`confidence_interval_upper = mean_difference + margin_of_error`
	`print("Margin of Error:", margin_of_error)`
	`print("95% Confidence Interval:", (confidence_interval_lower, confidence_interval_upper))`
		`# Print the results`
		`cat("t-Statistic:", t_statistic, "\n")`
		`cat("Degrees of Freedom:", degrees_freedom, "\n")`
		`cat("95% Confidence Interval for the difference:", conf_int[1], "to", conf_int[2], "\n")`
		`cat("Margin of Error:", (conf_int[2] - conf_int[1]) / 2, "\n")`

Estimated Parameter: Difference in population means $\mu_1 - \mu_2$

Sample Statistic: Difference in sample means $\bar{x}_1 - \bar{x}_2$

Confidence Interval Formula:

$$\bar{x}_1 - \bar{x}_2 \pm t_{\alpha/2} \times \widehat{S.E.}$$

$$\widehat{S.E.} = \sqrt{\frac{(n_1-1)s_1^2 + (n_2-1)s_2^2}{n_1+n_2-2}}$$

Assumptions:

The standard deviation for σ_1 and σ_2 is unknown

The samples are independent

The sample distributions for the two samples are approximately normal

The variance across the two samples is equal

```python
import numpy as np
from scipy import stats
# Sample data for two groups
group_1 = np.array([22, 25, 28, 30, 32])
group_2 = np.array([38, 40, 42, 45, 48])
# Calculate sample means and standard
deviations
mean_1 = np.mean(group_1)
mean_2 = np.mean(group_2)
std_dev_1 = np.std(group_1, ddof=1)
std_dev_2 = np.std(group_2, ddof=1)
# Calculate degrees of freedom for pooled
variance t-test
degrees_freedom = len(group_1) +
len(group_2) - 2
# Calculate pooled standard deviation
pooled_std_dev = np.sqrt(((len(group_1) -
1) * std_dev_1**2 + (len(group_2) - 1) *
std_dev_2**2) / degrees_freedom)
# Calculate t-score for a 95% confidence
interval
confidence_level = 0.95
t_score = stats.t.ppf((1 + confidence_
level) / 2, df=degrees_freedom)
# Calculate standard error of the
difference between means
standard_error_diff = pooled_std_dev *
np.sqrt(1/len(group_1) + 1/len(group_2))
# Calculate margin of error
margin_of_error = t_score *
standard_error_diff
```

```r
# Sample data for two groups
group_1 <- c(22, 25, 28, 30, 32)
group_2 <- c(38, 40, 42, 45, 48)
# Perform a two-sample t-test assuming
equal variances (pooled variance)
t_test_result <- t.test(group_1, group_2,
var.equal = TRUE, conf.level = 0.95)
# Extract the relevant values
mean_difference <- t_
test_result$estimate[1]
- t_test_result$estimate[2]
pooled_std_dev <- sqrt(t_test_
result$stderr^2) # Standard error used to
compute the pooled SD
degrees_freedom <- t_test_result$parameter
t_statistic <- t_test_result$statistic
conf_int <- t_test_result$conf.int
# Print the results
cat("Mean Difference:", mean_difference,
"\n")
cat("Pooled Standard Deviation:", pooled_
std_dev, "\n")
cat("Degrees of Freedom:", degrees_freedom,
"\n")
cat("t-Statistic:", t_statistic, "\n")
cat("95% Confidence Interval for the
difference:", conf_int[1], "to", conf_
int[2], "\n")
```

(Continued)

TABLE 4.2 (CONTINUED)

CI Type	Python Implementation	R Implementation

	```# Calculate confidence interval```
	 ```mean_difference = mean_1 - mean_2```
	 ```confidence_interval_lower = mean_difference```
	 ```- margin_of_error```
	 ```confidence_interval_upper = mean_difference```
	 ```+ margin_of_error```
	 ```print("Mean Difference:", mean_difference)```
	 ```print("Pooled Standard Deviation:",```
	 ```pooled_std_dev)```
	 ```print("Degrees of Freedom:",```
	 ```degrees_freedom)```
	 ```print("t-Score:", t_score)```
	 ```print("Standard Error of Difference:",```
	 ```standard_error_diff)```
	 ```print("Margin of Error:", margin_of_error)```
	 ```print("95% Confidence Interval:",```
	 ```(confidence_interval_lower,```
	 ```confidence_interval_upper))```	

Estimated Parameter:
 Paired difference population mean μ_d
 Sample Statistic:
 Paired difference sample mean $\bar{d}$
 Confidence Interval Formula:
 Paired difference
 $\bar{d} \pm t_{\alpha/2} \times \dfrac{s_d}{\sqrt{n}}$
	```import numpy as np```
	 ```from scipy import stats```
	 ```# Sample data for paired groups```
	 ```before = np.array([22, 25, 28, 30, 32])```
	 ```after = np.array([18, 20, 24, 25, 30])```
	 ```# Calculate the differences between paired```
	 ```observations```
	 ```differences = after - before```
	 ```# Calculate sample mean and standard error```
	 ```of the mean difference```
	 ```mean_diff = np.mean(differences)```
	 ```std_error_diff = stats.sem(differences)```
		```# Sample data for paired groups```
		 ```before <- c(22, 25, 28, 30, 32)```
		 ```after <- c(18, 20, 24, 25, 30)```
		 ```# Calculate the differences between paired```
		 ```observations```
		 ```differences <- after - before```
		 ```# Calculate sample mean and standard error```
		 ```of the mean difference```
		 ```mean_diff <- mean(differences)```
		 ```std_error_diff <- sd(differences) /```
		 ```sqrt(length(differences))```
		 ```# Calculate degrees of freedom```
		 ```degrees_freedom <- length(differences) - 1```
		 ```# Calculate t-score for a 95% confidence```
		 ```interval```

Assumptions:
The distribution of the differences is approximately equal
The number of pairs is ≥ 30

```python
# Calculate degrees of freedom
degrees_freedom = len(differences) - 1
# Calculate t-score for a 95% confidence interval
confidence_level = 0.95
t_score = stats.t.ppf((1 + confidence_level) / 2, df=degrees_freedom)
# Calculate margin of error
margin_of_error = t_score * std_error_diff
# Calculate confidence interval
confidence_interval_lower = mean_diff - margin_of_error
confidence_interval_upper = mean_diff + margin_of_error
print("Mean Difference:", mean_diff)
print("Standard Error of Difference:", std_error_diff)
print("Degrees of Freedom:", degrees_freedom)
print("t-Score:", t_score)
print("Margin of Error:", margin_of_error)
print("95% Confidence Interval:", (confidence_interval_lower, confidence_interval_upper))
```

```r
confidence_level <- 0.95
t_score <- qt((1 + confidence_level) / 2, df=degrees_freedom)
# Calculate margin of error
margin_of_error <- t_score * std_error_diff
# Calculate confidence interval
confidence_interval_lower <- mean_diff - margin_of_error
confidence_interval_upper <- mean_diff + margin_of_error
# Print results
cat("Mean Difference:", mean_diff, "\n")
cat("Standard Error of Difference:", std_error_diff, "\n")
cat("Degrees of Freedom:", degrees_freedom, "\n")
cat("t-Score:", t_score, "\n")
cat("Margin of Error:", margin_of_error, "\n")
cat("95% Confidence Interval: (", confidence_interval_lower, ", ", confidence_interval_upper, ")\n", sep="")
```

Estimated Parameter:
Population mean p
Sample Statistic:
Sample mean $\hat{p}$

```python
import statsmodels.api as sm
import statsmodels.stats.proportion as proportion
# Sample data
total_samples = 200
successes = 130
```

```r
# Sample data
total_samples <- 200
successes <- 130
# Calculate sample proportion
sample_proportion <- successes / total_samples
# Set confidence level
confidence_level <- 0.95
```

(Continued)

TABLE 4.2 (CONTINUED)

CI Type	Python Implementation	R Implementation
| Confidence Interval<br><br>Formula:<br><br>$\hat{p} \pm z_{\alpha/2}\sqrt{\dfrac{\hat{p}(1-\hat{p})}{n}}$<br><br>Assumptions:<br>Have at least ten successes and non-successes:<br><br>$n p_0 \geq 10 \; and \; n(1-p_0) \geq 10$ | ```
# Calculate sample proportion
sample_proportion = successes /
total_samples
# Set confidence level
confidence_level = 0.95
# Calculate confidence interval using
statsmodels
conf_interval = proportion.proportion_
confint(successes, total_samples, alpha=1-
confidence_level, method='normal')
# Display results
lower_bound, upper_bound = conf_interval
print(f"Sample Proportion:
{sample_proportion:.3f}")
print(f"Confidence Interval: ({lower_
bound:.3f}, {upper_bound:.3f})")
``` | ```
# Calculate standard error
std_error <- sqrt((sample_proportion *
(1 - sample_proportion)) / total_samples)
# Calculate z-score for the given
confidence level (95%)
z_score <- qnorm(1 - (1 - confidence_level)
/ 2)
# Calculate margin of error
margin_of_error <- z_score * std_error
# Calculate confidence interval
confidence_interval_lower <- sample_
proportion - margin_of_error
confidence_interval_upper <- sample_
proportion + margin_of_error
# Display results
cat("Sample Proportion:", round(sample_
proportion, 3), "\n")
cat("95% Confidence Interval: (",
round(confidence_interval_lower, 3), ", ",
round(confidence_interval_upper, 3), ")\n",
sep="")
``` |
| Estimated Parameter:<br>Population mean<br>$p_1 - p_2$<br>Sample Statistic:<br>Sample mean $\hat{p}_1 - \hat{p}_2$ | ```
import numpy as np
import statsmodels.api as sm
# Sample data for two proportions
successes_group_1 = 80
trials_group_1 = 100
successes_group_2 = 90
trials_group_2 = 120
# Calculate the confidence interval using
statsmodels' proportion_confint function
``` | |
```

Confidence Interval Formula:

$$\hat{p}_1 - \hat{p}_2 \pm z_{\alpha/2} \times \widehat{S.E.}$$

$$\widehat{S.E.} = \sqrt{\frac{\hat{p}_1(1-\hat{p}_1)}{n_1} + \frac{\hat{p}_2(1-\hat{p}_2)}{n_2}}$$

Assumptions:

Have at least ten successes and non-successes in each sample:

$$n_1 p_1, n_1(1-p_1), n_2 p_2, n_2(1-p_2) \geq 10$$

```
# This function automatically calculates
the confidence interval for a given
number of successes and trials
conf_interval_group_1 = sm.stats.
proportion_confint(successes_
group_1, trials_group_1, alpha=0.05,
method='normal')
conf_interval_group_2 = sm.stats.
proportion_confint(successes_
group_2, trials_group_2, alpha=0.05,
method='normal')
# Print results
print("Proportion Group 1:",
round(successes_group_1 / trials_group_1,
3))
print("Proportion Group 2:",
round(successes_group_2 / trials_group_2,
3))
print("95% Confidence Interval for Group
1:", conf_interval_group_1)
print("95% Confidence Interval for Group
2:", conf_interval_group_2)
# Calculate the difference in proportions
and the confidence interval for the
difference
diff_proportions = (successes_group_1 /
trials_group_1) - (successes_group_2 /
trials_group_2)
```

```
# Sample data for two proportions
successes_group_1 <- 80
trials_group_1 <- 100
successes_group_2 <- 90
trials_group_2 <- 120
# Combine successes and trials into vectors
successes <- c(successes_group_1,
successes_group_2)
trials <- c(trials_group_1, trials_group_2)
# Perform a two-proportion z-test using
prop.test()
test_result <- prop.test(successes, trials,
conf.level = 0.95)
# Print the results
cat("Proportion Group 1:", round(successes_
group_1 / trials_group_1, 3), "\n")
cat("Proportion Group 2:", round(successes_
group_2 / trials_group_2, 3), "\n")
cat("Difference in Proportions:",
round(test_result$estimate[1] - test_
result$estimate[2], 3), "\n")
cat("95% Confidence Interval for the
Difference:", test_result$conf.int, "\n")
```

(Continued)

TABLE 4.2 (CONTINUED)

CI Type	Python Implementation	R Implementation
| | ```
standard_error_diff = np.sqrt(
    (successes_group_1 * (1 - (successes_
group_1 / trials_group_1)) / trials_
group_1) +
    (successes_group_2 * (1 - (successes_
group_2 / trials_group_2)) /
trials_group_2)
)
z_score = sm.stats.proportion_confint(1,
1, alpha=0.05, method='normal')[1]
# Approximate z-score for 95% CI
margin_of_error = z_score *
standard_error_diff
confidence_interval_lower = diff_
proportions - margin_of_error
confidence_interval_upper = diff_
proportions + margin_of_error
# Print confidence interval for the
difference in proportions
print("Difference in Proportions:",
round(diff_proportions, 3))
print("95% Confidence Interval for the
Difference: (",
    round(confidence_interval_lower, 3), ",
    ",
    round(confidence_interval_upper, 3),
")")
``` | |
```

Additional Resources

Casella, G., & Berger, R. L. (2024). *Statistical Inference* (2nd ed.). Chapman & Hall/CRC Texts in Statistical Science.

Wasserman, L. (2010). *All of Statistics: A Concise Course in Statistical Inference* (Springer Texts in Statistics). Springer.

5

Regression Modeling

Invariably, newcomers to the field will struggle with deciding on an appropriate statistical model for their research question or business problem. In fact, it is one of the most common questions I'm asked by students, interns, and newly hired employees. Often, there is the perception that "more advanced" machine learning methods are necessary for credible analysis. In the search for an appropriate model, it is common to see what I call the *fumble-around-and-find-out* approach, where a host of statistical models is thrown at a problem without a clear rationale, including models such as random forests, XGBoost, convolutional neural networks, linear discriminant analysis, and support vector machines. The analyst then determines which model produces the most optimal or best-fit result based on a defined performance metric (yes, I'm looking at you, computer science majors). Another approach frequently used by newcomers (and even more seasoned analysts) is the fast abandonment of simple approaches in favor of more advanced machine learning models the moment that model assumptions are violated. For example, perhaps a multiple linear regression (we'll talk about this shortly) is fit to the data, and the analyst identifies some interaction between variables or a non-linear relationship between the predictor and response. In these cases, analysts often feel that they've reached the end of the road with regression and that machine learning models should be employed as the necessary next step (potentially sacrificing interpretability along the way).

While I appreciate the technical finesse required to implement these more sophisticated approaches, I suggest to newcomers to healthcare statistics in a world where we must explain our models to our clinical stakeholders that a more thoughtful ground-up method be considered where interpretability is favored over extreme optimization. When approaching a research question, I'll argue that the first question should be: What is the most straightforward and interpretable approach that appropriately addresses the research question (Occam's Razor)? As the analyst encounters difficulty with the simple model, incremental changes should be made to the model itself or the preparation of the variables. In this way, we prioritize interpretability and make surgical changes to the model to address specific data challenges.

DOI: 10.1201/9781003609759-5

This all might sound a bit nebulous, so let's ground this discussion in reality. This chapter will discuss regression, a modeling technique that allows us to generalize the relationship between a set of predictors and one or more response variables. Perhaps we're trying to estimate a patient's probability of a pressure ulcer (or bed sore)—a sore that results from prolonged pressure on a specific part of the body can develop in patients with extended hospital stays. The occurrence of a pressure ulcer would be the *response* (also called a dependent variable), and the patient characteristics would be the *predictors* (also called independent variables). Using language that is more specific to the healthcare problem, we could also say that the pressure ulcer is the *outcome*, and the patient characteristics are the *risk factors*. I tend to use the latter language when working on patient-level models but will switch between this terminology depending on context.

Regression models allow us to make predictions (such as the probability of a bed sore), but an equally important aspect of the model is how we interpret the association between the risk factors and the outcome. In some cases, we're not even interested in the resulting prediction; we use the model to understand how the various risk factors relate to an outcome (spoiler alert: we use hypothesis testing to do this).

The remainder of this chapter will be a guided tour of these models, and staying true to the motivation behind this book, we will discuss the conceptual justification for each model, the statistical notation, and an implemented example in Python and R. We'll spend more time discussing some models than others. I'll reiterate that in this book, we will not delve deep into the theory of each model, and the focus will be on the applied use of these models. That said, we do admittedly sacrifice depth for breadth to a certain degree. Additional resources have been provided at the end of this chapter for those interested in digging deeper into the theoretical minutia of a specific topic (and that, of course, is encouraged).

Figure 5.5 provides a beginner's road map for selecting a model based on the characteristics of the predictors and the response being evaluated. My intent with this figure is to show the range of regression implementations that allow common data scenarios to be addressed while preserving model interpretability.

Enough chitchat. Let's dig in.

Overview of Regression in Healthcare

Typically, we employ regression for two reasons. The first is to understand associations between predictor variables and a response variable. In this scenario, we interpret the resulting model *coefficients* to determine if there is a statistically significant association between the predictors and the response (or the risk factors and the outcome in the case of an outcome model).

When implementing regression to understand such associations, we must be extra careful when constructing the model and its unique data assumptions. We'll talk about model assumptions later in this chapter; however, as a representative example, one of the assumptions of regression modeling is that the predictor variables are independent. That is, two variables should not contain overlapping information (or at least be minimized). This can be a pesky task within clinical data as many clinical conditions are related. Perhaps we are building a model to predict a patient's length of stay. Among the many patient comorbidities in our model, we include the patient's liver disease diagnosis and self-reported alcohol use. If we were to evaluate the relationship between alcohol consumption and liver disease, we would find that the two conditions are generally correlated and, therefore, contain duplicative information content. Regression models will blindly optimize to produce a model that best fits the data. If two variables are highly correlated, our conclusions about the associations can be misleading. In such a scenario, the results of our hypothesis test (for the predictor variables) can result in a Type I error (we state that the association is not a result of chance) or a Type II error (we conclude that there is not an association when in fact there is). There are various ways to handle correlated data—with varying levels of sophistication. We'll discuss these options in more detail later in this chapter. The point is that we are playing a high-stakes game when using regression to identify clinical relationships. It cannot be overstated how important it is to carefully evaluate the data to ensure that the data conditions are appropriate for the employed model.

A second application of regression is to make a prediction or produce an expected value given the collective information we gather from the predictor variables. Perhaps we're building a model for a real-time decision support system, and we want to produce an alert to the care provider when a patient has a high risk of a fall (a common complication of inpatient care). In this case, we might emphasize the prediction's accuracy and place the coefficients' interpretability as a secondary focus. Of course, we do not want to understate the importance of interpreting the coefficients in a real-time model. When working with clinical stakeholders, they will want to know why an alert was fired for a given patient, and speaking from experience, stating that "the magic box produced this answer" will not be well received. We must balance the accuracy of the prediction while also being able to explain why the model produced a particular result.

Whether the motivation behind regression modeling is to make predictions or to understand some association between predictors and responses, we will generally use the same core set of tools. Let's open this toolbox and explore some of its contents.

We can group the most salient forms of regression into two categories— ordinary least squares (OLS) regression and generalized linear models (GLMs). Technically, OLS is a form of GLM, but let's not make this more confusing than needed.

We'll cover OLS models and GLMs in the paragraphs below, but for now, it's important to know that OLS models are used for modeling continuous outcomes and can fit with a "closed form" solution. That is, a single equation using matrix algebra (yuck) can produce the fitted model. We must leverage more sophisticated methods to address more complex data scenarios—such as modeling outcomes with non-normal distributions. GLMs allow us to model more complex data scenarios but require an iterative form of optimization (often using a process called "maximum likelihood estimation" [MLE]). Luckily, our friends in the open-source community have made available several statistical packages that abstract away this complexity, and from an implementation perspective, an OLS and GLM are nearly identical in Python and R.

I prefer problem-based learning rather than simply cataloging the various forms of regression. Therefore, in the following sections, we'll discuss OLS models and GLMs based on the type of problem they solve. For example, we'll discuss logistic regression under the header "Modeling Binary Outcomes". This way, the reader will not have to sift through the various models to identify the one most suited to their research problem.

There are, of course, a number of data scenarios where basic forms of OLS and GLMs will be insufficient. The next chapter is the statistical equivalent of "break this glass in case of an emergency". Here, we will introduce the next level of sophistication to handle more complex data scenarios. These models are typically reserved for graduate-level courses; however, given the prevalence of the data problems in healthcare data that these models address, it is important that we dedicate time to them. Here, we will introduce generalized additive models (my favorite secret weapon in statistics), zero-inflated models (for pesky scenarios where we have lots of zeros alongside a continuous distribution), and a host of other model types and methods.

Ordinary Least Squares Regression

Linear regression models are designed to generalize a linear relationship between one or more predictor variables and a continuous response variable. *Simple* linear regression refers to models that use one predictor variable, while *multiple* (or "multivariable") linear regression refers to models using multiple predictor variables.

Let's start with the most basic examples using a simple linear regression. We have a response variable (systolic blood pressure) and a predictor variable (patient age), and we want to estimate the response variable based on our predictor variable. The data for this simple model is shown in Figure 5.1. This mock data shows a linear relationship between age and BMI for adults 18–65. Suppose we position a line to the data points to minimize the collective distance between all the data points and the line. In that case, we (conceptually) fit a model whereby the linear relationship between age and BMI is quantified through the slope of the line and its intersection with the y-axis.

This optimization process is called OLS, which involves minimizing the sum of squared residuals (i.e., the sum of the squared distances between the data point and the line). You might recall the slope of a line as $y = mx + b$ in your middle school math class. Statisticians like to jazz things up a bit, and so this formula is generally written as follows:

$$Y = \alpha + \beta_1 X_1 + \varepsilon$$

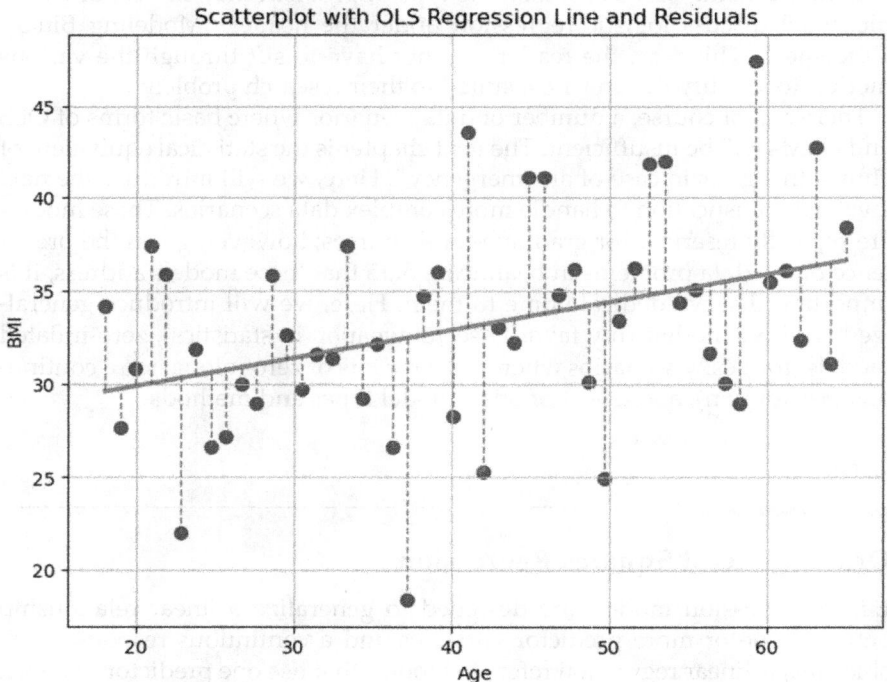

Scatterplot with OLS Regression Line and Residuals

FIGURE 5.1
Ordinary Least Squares (OLS) fit optimized by minimizing the sum of squared residuals.

where

> Y is the dependent variable (BMI). It is the value that we are trying to estimate through the combination of predictor variables. In the case of simple linear regression, we have one predictor variable (age).
>
> α represents the intercept, which we can define as the estimated response variable when all predictor variables are set to zero, providing a starting point for the linear relationship between the predictor and the response. In the BMI example, it would be the expected BMI when age = 0.
>
> β_1 is the coefficient (think about the slope of a line) that quantifies the relationships between age and systolic blood pressure. In this hypothetical example, each unit increase in the patient's age is associated with an β_1 increase in BMI.
>
> ε represents the error term, which accounts for unexplained variation in BMI that is not captured by the linear relationship with age. Many other factors may help us explain changes in a person's BMI, such as their diet, activity level, genetic characteristics, disability, and disease status. The error term ε represents the error in our estimation of Y due to unaccounted-for variables in our model that help explain Y. All models will have some degree of error. We aim to minimize that error by including a holistic set of variables that help us explain the outcome. In generalizing a model, there will always be some degree of error, as we cannot capture all the factors that might explain some outcome.

Disclaimer: This model is for demonstration only, and there are issues with modeling age and BMI as a linear relationship, as the relationship between age and BMI will be nonlinear across various stages of aging.

Regression equations can be expressed in a variety of ways. For example, we might write the same equation as $y = \beta_0 + \beta_1 X_1$, where β_0 is the intercept value, or in a way that is specific to our research question, B $MI = \alpha + \beta_1$ Age. It is always best to be as explicit as possible with notation so that there is less onus on the reader to decipher potentially cryptic notation. While flexing your statistical muscles with elaborate calligraphic notation is tempting, you are more likely to receive buy-in from clinical stakeholders if the approach can be easily interpreted.

Recall that one use of regression is interpreting the coefficients. Let's examine the model statistics for our predictor variable, BMI, in the BMI example (Table 5.1).

What a mess this is! Take a deep breath. We'll get through this together.

In the first column, we have *const*, which represents a constant (i.e., the intercept value). This variable is α the point at which the line intersects

TABLE 5.1

Example Coefficient Results From a Simple Linear Regression Model

	coef	std. err	t	$p > \lvert t \rvert$	[0.025	0.975]
const	26.935	2.386	11.29	0	22.138	31.732
x1	0.1498	0.055	2.747	0.008	0.04	0.259

TABLE 5.2

Example Coefficient Results from a Multivariable Linear Regression Model

	coef	std. error	t	$p > \lvert t \rvert$	[0.025	0.975]
const	25.6964	1.016	25.302	0	23.681	27.712
Age	0.4687	0.02	23.903	0	0.43	0.508
Sex	1.2305	0.402	3.062	0.003	0.433	2.028
Activity	−1.8132	0.212	−8.552	0	−2.234	−1.392

with the y-axis. It's the starting point of our model before adjusting for the various predictors. The $x1$ value represents the predictor variable (age in our example), and its coeff value represents the slope of the line from Table 5.2. As we add additional variables to the model, they will be listed as $X_1, \ldots, X_n$.

Just when you thought we were done with hypothesis testing and confidence intervals, they are back! The remaining columns in this table involve specific hypothesis tests for the intercept and coefficient values.

For the intercept value (const), our null hypothesis is that the intercept is zero, and the alternate hypothesis is that it is not zero. While this is useful information, the most noteworthy information involves interpreting the coefficients for the individual predictors. In the case of our predictor variable (age), here labeled as x1, we are testing the null hypothesis that the slope of the line is zero and the alternate hypothesis that the slope of the coefficient is not zero. In other words, we are testing that the linear relationship between the predictor variable and the response variable is not likely to be by chance (when accounting for all other variables in the model).

In each of these testing scenarios (the intercept and the individual predictors), we are given the standard error (std. err), t-statistic (t), two-tailed p-value ($p > \lvert t \rvert$), and the 95% confidence values in which the true intercept or coefficient (i.e., slope) exists. The 0.025 and 0.975 columns, therefore, represent the lower 95% confidence interval. Recall that since this is a two-tailed test, the significance level is divided by two such that .025 (or 2.5%) of the data is represented at each tail.

In linear regression, interpreting the coefficients is easy. We can say that each unit increase in age (or $x1$) is associated with β_1 an increase in BMI (or *y*). Notice that we are being careful with our words here. We do not want to imply that there is a causal relationship, so it is generally good practice to use words like "associate" rather than "causes" or "results in".

There is a specific and quickly growing field of statistics called "causal inference", where statistical models are designed to identify causality. This field of statistics is fascinating, and many of the techniques discussed in this book are foundational concepts that will be useful for someone interested in causal analysis. However, we will not discuss causal inference in depth.

Now that we have a fitted model, we can apply it to new observations (i.e., patients outside the sample we used to fit our model). For example, I am 45 years old (stop laughing), and using this crude model fitted using mock data, we can use the intercept value and age coefficient to estimate or predict my BMI.

$$33.676 = 26.935 + \left(45 \, x \, 0.1498 \right)$$

Even if we used actual observed patient data for this model, it would undoubtedly produce abysmal results. That is, of course, because we are using minimal information about the patient. If only there were a way to use more information about the patient to estimate their BMI. Well, you guessed it—there is! Using multiple linear regression, we can account for multiple patient characteristics and reduce the error in our prediction.

Multiple Linear Regression

In multiple linear regression, we use more than one variable to estimate the outcome. We could update our model to include body mass index (BMI). That model can be written as follows:

$$\text{BMI} = \alpha + \beta_1 \, \text{Age}_1 + \beta_2 \, \text{Sex}_2 + \beta_3 \, \text{Activity Level}_3 + \varepsilon$$

Or, more generally, this can be written as follows:

$$Y = \alpha + \beta_1 X_1 + \ldots + \beta_n X_n + \varepsilon$$

The interpretation of a simple linear regression is, well ... simple. The relationship between the response and a predictor variable is a straight line. If we include an additional variable, the model can be conceptualized as a plane in three-dimensional coordinate space. With the third variable and any additional predictor beyond two, we end up with a hyperplane across n-dimensions. Practically speaking, however, it is important to know that the relationship between each predictor variable and the response (symbolized as β_i) quantifies the association between a single predictor and an outcome when all other variables are held constant.

Using the BMI example above, let's look at a multiple linear regression in Python.

```python
import numpy as np
import pandas as pd
import statsmodels.api as sm
np.random.seed(0)
n = 100  # Number of samples
age = np.random.normal(40, 10, n)
sex = np.random.choice([0, 1], n)  # 0 for female, 1 for
male
activity_levels = np.random.normal(3, 1, n)
bmi = 25 + 0.5 * age + 1.5 * sex - 2 * activity_levels +
np.random.normal(0, 2, n)
pat_data_df = pd.DataFrame({'Age': age, 'Sex': sex,
'Activity': activity_levels, 'BMI': bmi})
X = pat_data_df[['Age', 'Sex', 'Activity']]
X = sm.add_constant(X)
y = pat_data_df['BMI']
model = sm.OLS(y, X).fit()
print(model.summary())
```

In this example, we use the `statsmodels` package to fit an OLS model `sm.OLS(y, X).fit()`. The constant term `sm.add_constant(X)` is necessary to ensure that an intercept value is included in the model.

If we peek at the coefficient summary from our model, we can see that increased activity is negatively associated with BMI—as activity increases, BMI decreases. We can also see that BMI increases with age and that males are slightly more likely to have a higher BMI. Each variable is significant at the 95% confidence level since it is below .05.

Using R, the implementation might look like this:

```r
library(broom)
n <- 100  # Number of samples
age <- rnorm(n, mean = 40, sd = 10)
sex <- sample(c(0, 1), n, replace = TRUE)  # 0 for
female, 1 for male
activity_levels <- rnorm(n, mean = 3, sd = 1)
bmi <- 25 + 0.5 * age + 1.5 * sex - 2 * activity_levels +
rnorm(n, mean = 0, sd = 2)
pat_data_df <- data.frame(Age = age, Sex = sex, Activity
= activity_levels, BMI = bmi)
pat_bmi_model <- lm(BMI ~ Age + Sex + Activity, data =
pat_data_df)
summary(pat_bmi_model)
tidy(pat_bmi_model)
```

Here, we use the `lm` function to run a linear model (an OLS model). The tidy function from the `broom` package is used to format the coefficients into a two-by-two data frame similar to the table shown in Table 5.2. I highly recommend the broom package for extracting model coefficients (a well as performance statistics and other model metadata).

Generalized Linear Models

And now for my favorite subject—GLMs. GLMs, the Swiss army knife of interpretable modeling, are based on a flexible model framework that allows us to swap out its component parts to solve a wide range of data problems. Like OLS models, GLMs allow us to model the relationship between a response variable and one or more predictor variables; however, GLMs can additionally be used to model outcomes with strong rightward skew (long tails to the right), as we commonly see with cost and length of stay data, binary outcomes such as mortality and readmissions, or nominal outcomes (where a variety of outcomes are possible), such as complications (of course they can be binary too). We can certainly model normal distributions with a GLM as well. In fact, an OLS model and a GLM will produce the same results, as an OLS model is technically a type of GLM. Any distribution that falls within the *exponential family* of distributions can be modeled—providing that we use the proper components.

When a new data problem is put in front of me (where response and predictors are involved), my first thought is, "Can I use a GLM for this?" Case in point: Of the 20 published papers I've authored or coauthored in the last three years, 17 have used some form of GLMs to address a wide range of healthcare-related issues.

There are three primary components in a GLM: (1) the linear predictor, (2) the probability distribution, and (3) the link function.

First is the *probability distribution* itself. Here, we are specifically talking about the distribution of the response variable. If we were to plot the response variable distribution as a histogram, we should be able to naturally intuit the distribution of the data (or at least narrow the candidate list). By picking the distribution, we are defining the distributional characteristics of the outcome to ensure that predictors are optimized in the context of that distribution and that the resulting predictions are constrained to the shape of the designated distribution. Common distributions include the Gaussian (normal) distribution for continuous data, the binomial distribution for binary data, and the Poisson distribution for count data. Other important distributions are the negative binomial, gamma, and exponential distributions. We'll focus on examples common to specific health outcomes; however, it is important to understand that the framework can be adapted to problems outside the specific examples here.

Next is the *linear predictor*, which, as we saw in the OLS example, is a function of the linear combination of the predictor variables. That is, the intercept value and predictor variables are weighted by their respective coefficients (i.e., $\alpha + \beta_1 x_1 + \beta_2 x_2 + \ldots + \beta_n x_n$). The linear predictor is typically represented by the Greek character η (eta) as shown in the below notation:

$$\eta = \alpha + \beta_1 x_1 + \beta_2 x_2 + \cdots + \beta_n x_n$$

The linear combination of predictors η is an unbounded function. The result can be positive or negative, depending on the values of the predictors, and there are no constraints in the resulting value. If we want to model a binary outcome, for example, nothing prevents the result from producing a value outside the range of 0 to 1. We certainly don't want our model to produce a negative value or a value greater than 1.

How, then, do we relate the unique nature of the outcome distribution to the linear combination of predictors? Well, the link function, that is! (Come on. I'm trying to sound excited about this). The link function allows us to model the outcome linearly despite the unique shape of the target distribution. In the case of a binary outcome, the link function allows us to relate a binary outcome to a linear predictor. As we can see in the formula below, the link function allows us to model the probability of an event using a *logit* link function.

$$\eta = ln\left(\frac{P}{1-P}\right) = \alpha + \beta_1 X_1 + \ldots + \beta_n X_n$$

Here, we see that the linear combination of variables η represents the log odds $ln\left(\dfrac{P}{1-P}\right)$ of the probability. We cannot use the linear combination of variables to produce a probability, but we can model the log-odds (using a "natural log").

The resulting value η can subsequently be transformed into a probability p, properly bounded between 0 and 1 using the appropriate inverse link function (in this case, the sigmoid function). We represent the inverse link function more generally as g.

$$p = g(\eta) = \frac{1}{1+e^{-\eta}}$$

Table 5.3 provides a quick guide to the link function and inverse link function most frequently used for Gaussian, Poisson, and Binomial distributions, which are common within healthcare.

Wowzers Mike. I'm still confused.

Okay, let me summarize. A GLM consists of three fundamental components: the probability distribution, the linear predictor, and the link function. The choice of a probability distribution is necessary to match the data's characteristics, with common options like Gaussian for continuous data, Poisson for rightward skewed distributions (especially when count data is being modeled), and binomial for binary outcomes (see Table 5.3). The linear predictor combines the predictor variables, but it can produce unbounded values, necessitating the link function. The link function acts like a translator by turning the unlimited values from the linear combination of predictors into predictions that make sense for our data, such as keeping probabilities between 0 and 1 or making sure counts aren't negative. Once the data is modeled linearly (with the help of the link function), the data can be converted back to its original scale with the inverse link function. In the case of a binary outcome, we used the *logit* link function to model a binary outcome as log odds and the *sigmoid* inverse link function to convert those log odds back into probabilities. By understanding and combining these components, GLMs provide a versatile framework for modeling a wide range of data types.

TABLE 5.3

Canonical and Inverse Link Functions by Response Distribution for Linear, Logistic, and Poisson GLMs

Type of Regression	When to Use	Probability Distribution	Canonical Link Function	Inverse Link Function
Linear Regression	When modeling continuous outcomes with a linear relationship between predictors and the response.	Gaussian (Normal)	Identity Link $\eta = \mu$	$g(\eta) = \eta$
Logistic Regression	When modeling binary or categorical outcomes (mortality, complications, readmissions)	Binomial	Logit Link $\eta = \log\left(\dfrac{\mu}{1-\mu}\right)$	$g(\eta) = \dfrac{1}{1+e^{-\eta}}$
Poisson Regression	When modeling count data or event rates where the response variable follows a Poisson distribution (cost, charge, LOS)	Poisson	Log Link $\eta = \log(\mu)$	$g(\eta) = e^{\eta}$

We've done some hand-waiving here regarding the optimization of GLMs which are fit through an iterative process whereby the parameter estimates (β) are adjusted incrementally to produce the optimal model fit. This is commonly done through a process called MLE, although other optimization methods can be used. We won't dig too deep into MLE and the concept of likelihood. It is important to know that the link function is critical in this optimization process because it transforms the model structure into a linear form, allowing for efficient estimation of the model coefficients.

In the following chapters, we'll provide some applied examples of GLMs. In keeping with this book's goal, the statistical notation will be provided alongside the Python and R code for each data scenario. Note that a more generic statistical notation has been provided in the following paragraphs for consistency across distributions (and to demonstrate GLMs as a unified framework); however, alternative notation for each of the three primary models discussed below has also been provided in Table 5.4. The notation in this table is more common when writing about specific models (e.g., a logistic regression) and would be my recommended notation if writing about the model in a white paper or publication. Table 5.4 also provides a snippet of Python and R code to show the notation and implementation side by side.

Selecting an Appropriate Model

In most scenarios, our research question involves understanding how a set of predictor variables is associated with a continuous or categorical response variable. Continuous response variables can be normal or skewed in some way. Categorical variables can have a single category, such as the binary occurrence of mortality, or multiple categories (e.g., complications occurring in the hospital).

Modeling Continuous Data

Continuous data can come in many shapes (or distributions), which, as we have discussed previously, will determine the most appropriate model to fit our predictors. In this section, we'll cover two primary data scenarios: normally distributed data and rightward skewed data.

TABLE 5.4

Regression Notation and Examples

Regression Model	Regression Model Details	Example	Description
Linear Regression	Response Distribution	$Y \sim \mathcal{N}(\mu, \sigma^2)$	Models continuously have outcomes with a normal distribution. $\mathcal{N}(\mu, \sigma^2)$ indicates that the response is normally distributed with a mean μ and a constant variance σ^2
	Functional Form	$\mu = \alpha + \beta_1 x_1 + \dots + \beta_{p-1} x_{p-1}$	A linear relationship between predictors and the response gives the estimated mean response μ.
	Python Implementation	`from sklearn.linear_model import LinearRegressionmodel = LinearRegression().fit(X, y)`	Use LinearRegression from scikit-learn for fitting the model.
	R Implementation	`linear_mod <- glm(y ~ ., data = df)`	Use glm() function with the default family as Gaussian to fit a linear model.
Logistic Regression	Response Distribution	$Y \sim \text{Ber}(P)$	Models binary or categorical outcomes with a Bernoulli distribution. P represents the probability of the response being 1 (success).
	Functional Form	$\log\left(\frac{P}{1=P}\right) = \alpha + \beta_1 x_1 + \dots + \beta_{p-1} x_{p-1}$	The logit link function models the log-odds of the probability as a linear combination of predictors.
	Python Implementation	`from sklearn.linear_model import LogisticRegressionmodel = LogisticRegression().fit(X, y)`	Use LogisticRegression from scikit-learn to fit the logistic model.
	R Implementation	`logistic_mod <- glm(y ~ ., family = binomial(), data = df)`	Use glm() with the binomial() family to fit a logistic regression model.

(Continued)

TABLE 5.4 (CONTINUED)

Regression Model	Regression Model Details	Example	Description
Poisson Regression	Response Distribution	$Y \sim \text{Poisson}(\mu)$	Models count data or event rates with a Poisson distribution, where μ is the mean count.
	Functional Form	$\log(\mu) = \alpha + \beta_1 x_1 + \ldots + \beta_{p-1} x_{p-1}$	The log link function models the log of the mean response μ as a linear combination of the predictors.
	Python Implementation	`from sklearn.linear_model import PoissonRegression` `model = PoissonRegression().fit(X, y)`	Use PoissonRegression from sklearn (or statsmodels for more flexibility) to fit the Poisson model.
	R Implementation	`poisson_mod <- glm(y ~ ., family = poisson(), data = df)`	Use glm() with the poisson() family to fit a Poisson regression model.

Modeling Normal Distributions

In the above section on OLS, an example model was provided with BMI as the dependent variable and age, sex, and activity level as predictor variables. Providing the same dataset, the OLS and GLM will produce the same results, and we will represent the model using the same notation.

$$\text{BMI} = \alpha + \beta_1 \text{Age}_1 + \beta_2 \text{Sex}_2 + \beta_3 \text{Activity Level}_3 + \varepsilon$$

Or more generally

$$Y = \alpha + \beta_1 X_1 + \cdots + \beta_n X_n + \varepsilon$$

Given that the distribution is normal and can be modeled directly through the linear combination of predictors, no transformation is needed for the link function (and, therefore, the inverse link function). Technically, we use the *identity* link function, but no transformation is required. The identity link function directly models the expected value of the response variable based on the linear combination of predictor variables without changing or transforming it.

An implementation of the same research question demonstrated using OLS above is shown below using a GLM model with normal or "Gaussian" distribution:

```
import numpy as np
import pandas as pd
import statsmodels.api as sm
np.random.seed(0)
n = 100   # Number of samples
age = np.random.normal(40, 10, n)
sex = np.random.choice([0, 1], n)   # 0 for female, 1 for
male
activity_levels = np.random.normal(3, 1, n)
bmi = 25 + 0.5 * age + 1.5 * sex - 2 * activity_levels +
np.random.normal(0, 2, n)
data = pd.DataFrame({'Age': age, 'Sex': sex, 'Activity':
activity_levels, 'BMI': bmi})
X = data[['Age', 'Sex', 'Activity']]
X = sm.add_constant(X)
y = data['BMI']
glm_model = sm.GLM(y, X, family=sm.families.Gaussian()).
fit()
print(glm_model.summary())
```

Notice that, in this example, the model is fit using `sm.GLM(y, X, family=sm.families.Gaussian()).fit()` rather than the OLS function `sm.OLS(y, X).fit()`. This shows that we are using the larger GLM framework, specifying a normal or "Gaussian" distribution. The GLM class in statsmodels will select the "canonical" link function for us that is appropriate for the selected distribution (Table 5.3)

In this model, the coefficients indicate the change in the original response variable for a one-unit increase in the corresponding predictor variable. A positive coefficient suggests that a unit increase in the predictor variable is associated with an increase in the response variable by a quantity of β, assuming a constant proportional effect. For example, if the coefficient is 0.1, it implies a .01 increase in the response variable for every one-unit increase in the predictor variable.

Likewise in R, we can implement a GLM with a Gaussian distribution in a similar manner, passing in the gaussian() function call as an argument to the glm function:

```
set.seed(0)
n <- 100   # Number of samples
age <- rnorm(n, mean = 40, sd = 10)
sex <- sample(c(0, 1), n, replace = TRUE)   # 0 for
female, 1 for male
activity_levels <- rnorm(n, mean = 3, sd = 1)
bmi <- 25 + 0.5 * age + 1.5 * sex - 2 * activity_levels +
rnorm(n, mean = 0, sd = 2)
data <- data.frame(Age = age, Sex = sex, Activity =
activity_levels, BMI = bmi)
glm_model <- glm(BMI ~ Age + Sex + Activity, data = data,
family = gaussian())
summary(glm_model)
```

Modeling Skewed Distributions: Using Log Transformation

Rightward-skewed data is common in healthcare, especially with count-based outcomes such as LOS, cost, and charge. Several regression modeling options are available when working with data where the response variable is rightward skewed (i.e., has a longer tail to the right).

The first is to use a true linear model that assumes a normal distribution. This can be an OLS model or GLM (remember, they produce the same results). The trick here is that we first apply a log transformation to the response variable so that the distribution is coerced (hopefully) into a normal distribution. A visual inspection of the distribution before and after transformation will often be sufficient to determine if the data distribution is log-normal (i.e., normal when the log is transformed). There are more formal tests of normality (e.g., Shapiro-Wilk, Anderson-Darling, and Kolmogorov-Smirnov tests) if additional rigor is needed in your analysis.

Log transformations gracefully compress data so that more extreme values near the tail are pulled toward the center—making log modeling an appropriate choice for skewed data. Another benefit to the log transformation is that outliers generally become less influential since the scale of the data is compressed through the log transformation. We might express a model fit to patient length of stay as follows:

$$log(Y) = \alpha + \beta_1 X_1 + \ldots + \beta_n X_n + \varepsilon$$

Since we are force-fitting the response variable into a normal distribution, no link function is required.

Let's suppose we are estimating the cost of an inpatient stay, data typically distributed with rightward skew. To employ a log model, we would transform the total cost for each patient stay with a log transformation (i.e., log(cost)) and use the log cost as the response variable in our linear model.

Python

```
import pandas as pd
import statsmodels.api as sm
import numpy as np
data = {
    'cost': [1000, 1200, 800, 1500, 2000, 900, 1100,
1700, 950, 1300],
    'age': [45, 32, 67, 54, 21, 38, 49, 60, 27, 40],
    'sex': [1, 0, 1, 0, 1, 0, 1, 0, 1, 0],  # 1 for male,
0 for female
    'covid_indicator': [1, 0, 0, 1, 1, 0, 0, 1, 1, 0],  #
1 for COVID, 0 for no COVID
}
df = pd.DataFrame(data)
df['log_cost'] = np.log(df['cost'])
X = df[['age', 'sex', 'covid_indicator']]
X = sm.add_constant(X)  # Add a constant (intercept) term
to the model
y = df['log_cost']
lognormal_model = sm.GLM(y, X, family=sm.families.
Gaussian()).fit()
print(lognormal_model.summary())
```

R

```
data <- data.frame(
   cost = c(1000, 1200, 800, 1500, 2000, 900, 1100, 1700,
950, 1300),
   age = c(45, 32, 67, 54, 21, 38, 49, 60, 27, 40),
   sex = c(1, 0, 1, 0, 1, 0, 1, 0, 1, 0),  # 1 for male, 0
for female
   covid_indicator = c(1, 0, 0, 1, 1, 0, 0, 1, 1, 0)  # 1
for COVID, 0 for no COVID
   )
```

```
data$log_cost <- log(data$cost)
lognormal_model <- glm(log_cost ~ age + sex + covid_
indicator, data = data, family = gaussian())
summary(lognormal_model)
```

As shown in the example above, our response variable (cost) is transformed using the numpy log function np.log() or simply log() in R. The model is then fit to the predictor variables.

It is important to note that we have specified a normal or "Gaussian" distribution as the GLM distribution and simply applied a pre-processing step to transform the response variable to a normal distribution.

Additionally, our predicted values from this model will also be on a log scale, and we must exponentiate (i.e., apply the antilog) to convert the prediction back to the original cost scale.

Note that due to the log transformation of the response variable, the scale of the model coefficients is also on a log scale. For example, a unit step increase in age (i.e., a year) is associated with a β increase in the log cost. For improved interpretability, we can exponentiate the coefficient such that $\exp(\beta)$ represents the increase in the response variable (i.e., cost) with each unit increase in X (i.e., age) when all other variables are held constant.

Note that the log of zero results in infinity; therefore, a log transformation applied to zero values can result in errors in the code. One way to handle this is to add 1 to all values before the log transformation. Just as we add 1 before the log transformation, we must also subtract 1 from the exponentiated values when converting the prediction back to its original scale.

Modeling Skewed Distributions: Using Poisson Regression (and other distributions)

Arguably, a more elegant solution for modeling outcomes with rightward skew is to use a GLM with an appropriate distribution. For example, cost, charge, and length of stay outcomes are based on the count of days or dollars and will naturally have a rightward skew. These variables start at zero (or 1) and are distributed such that the bulk of the data is near the left-hand side of the distribution, with a long tail of more extreme values. Within a particular disease group, most patients will have a length of stay in a similar range; however, there will be exceptional patients with a longer LOS due to the complexity of their diagnoses or operational challenges (no place to discharge the patient). The same will be true with the cost of an inpatient stay or episode, where some smaller proportion of the patient population will have more extreme costs due to specialized treatment.

While we could log transform the response variables to coerce the data into a more normal distribution, a GLM model allows us to model the distribution outright by specifying a distribution that naturally aligns with the distribution of the outcome. A Poisson model is generally a good starting point for cost data, as a count of dollars (although Gamma or Negative binomial distributions should also be considered). The Poisson distribution uses the log link function as shown as follows:

$$\eta = log(\lambda) = \alpha + \beta_1 X_1 + \ldots + \beta_n X_n$$

where λ represents the expected rate of occurrence of the dependent variable.

Given that the log link function is used for the Poisson distribution (Table 5.3), the model's resulting values can be converted back to their original scale through exponentiation (the antilog), the inverse link function.

$$g(\eta) = e^\eta$$

While the log-transformed linear model and Poisson model appear similar structurally—in that, the linear combination of the predictor variables is exponentiated to obtain a prediction on the scale of the original distribution—the models are fit in quite different ways. Unlike the log-transformed model, no log transformation is applied to the response variable itself in Poisson regression. The Poisson distribution inherently models count data. As such, no special handling in the Poisson model is needed to account for potential zero values in the distribution.

Python

```
import pandas as pd
import statsmodels.api as sm
import numpy as np
data = {
    'cost': [1000, 1200, 800, 1500, 2000, 900, 1100,
1700, 950, 1300],
    'age': [45, 32, 67, 54, 21, 38, 49, 60, 27, 40],
    'sex': [1, 0, 1, 0, 1, 0, 1, 0, 1, 0],   # 1 for male,
0 for female
    'covid_indicator': [1, 0, 0, 1, 1, 0, 0, 1, 1, 0],   #
1 for COVID, 0 for no COVID
}
df = pd.DataFrame(data)
X = df[['age', 'sex', 'covid_indicator']]
X = sm.add_constant(X)   # Add a constant (intercept) term
to the model
y = df['cost']
poisson_model = sm.GLM(y, X, family=sm.families.
Poisson()).fit()
```

```
predicted_cost = poisson_model.predict(X)
print(poisson_model.summary())
```

R

```
data <- data.frame(
  cost = c(1000, 1200, 800, 1500, 2000, 900, 1100, 1700,
950, 1300),
  age = c(45, 32, 67, 54, 21, 38, 49, 60, 27, 40),
  sex = c(1, 0, 1, 0, 1, 0, 1, 0, 1, 0),  # 1 for male, 0
for female
  covid_indicator = c(1, 0, 0, 1, 1, 0, 0, 1, 1, 0)  # 1
for COVID, 0 for no COVID
)
poisson_model <- glm(cost ~ age + sex + covid_indicator,
data = data, family = poisson())
predicted_cost <- predict(poisson_model, type =
"response")
summary(poisson_model)
```

Here, we can see that the Poisson distribution is specified in the GLM rather than a Gaussian distribution in the previous example. In Python, we use `family = sm.families.Poisson()`, while, in R, we similarly use `family = poisson()`. The outcome is modeled for us directly using the appropriate link function (which, again, these functions are doing for us with their canonical defaults). These functions do provide an option to override the link function if desired.

In Poisson regression, the coefficients represent the effect on the expected count of occurrences for a one-unit change in the predictor variable, while holding other predictors constant. For example, if β_1 is 0.1, this implies that for every one-unit increase in x_1, the expected count increases by a factor of exp(0.1), which is approximately 1.105. In other words, the expected count is approximately 10.5% higher for each one-unit increase in X1.

There are scenarios where other data distributions may be more appropriate. For example, the negative binomial and gamma distributions may also be considered and can provide a better fit depending on the unique characteristics of the data.

Modeling Binary Outcomes

Suppose we want to model a binary outcome, like inpatient mortality, based on a set of patient characteristics. If we use the OLS approach, our model is likely to produce values outside the boundaries of our observed distributions—that is, the values could be less than zero (negative) or greater than one. A more appropriate model would be logistic regression, a member of the GLM family of models.

We cannot derive a binary outcome from a linear combination of predictors, as no constraint exists to prevent the resulting value from being outside the range of probabilities (0 to 1). Therefore, the linear combination of predictors is fit to the log-odds of the probabilities (i.e., the logit link function). This allows the linear combination of predictors to produce a real number that is not bounded between 0 and 1.

$$\eta = ln\left(\frac{P}{1-P}\right) = \alpha + \beta_1 X_1 + ... + \beta_n X_n$$

The *sigmoid* inverse link function can be applied to the linear combination of predictors to reshape the result into probability p, naturally bounded between 0 and 1.

$$g(\eta) = \frac{1}{1+e^{-\eta}}$$

Let's consider a scenario where we are interested in the association between a set of patient characteristics (age, biological sex, COVID-19, and diabetes) and mortality using a sample of acute inpatient stays:

Python

```
import statsmodels.api as sm
import pandas as pd
data = {
    'age': [45, 32, 67, 54, 21, 38, 49, 60, 27, 40],
    'sex': [1, 0, 1, 0, 1, 0, 1, 0, 1, 0],  # 1 for male,
0 for female
    'covid_indicator': [1, 0, 0, 1, 1, 0, 0, 1, 1, C],  #
1 for COVID, 0 for no COVID
    'diabetes_indicator': [0, 1, 0, 1, 0, 0, 1, 0, 1, 0],
# 1 for diabetes, 0 for no diabetes
    'mortality': [1, 0, 1, 1, 0, 1, 0, 1, 1, 0]  # 1 for
yes, 0 for no
}
df = pd.DataFrame(data)
X = sm.add_constant(df[['age', 'sex', 'covid_indicator',
'diabetes_indicator']])
logistic_model = sm.GLM(df['mortality'], X, family=sm.
families.Binomial()).fit()
print(logistic_model.summary())
```

R

```
data <- data.frame(
  age = c(45, 32, 67, 54, 21, 38, 49, 60, 27, 40),
  sex = c(1, 0, 1, 0, 1, 0, 1, 0, 1, 0),  # 1 for male, 0
for female
  covid_indicator = c(1, 0, 0, 1, 1, 0, 0, 1, 1, 0),  # 1
for COVID, 0 for no COVID
  diabetes_indicator = c(0, 1, 0, 1, 0, 0, 1, 0, 1, 0),
# 1 for diabetes, 0 for no diabetes
  mortality = c(1, 0, 1, 1, 0, 1, 0, 1, 1, 0)  # 1 for
yes, 0 for no
)
logistic_model <- glm(mortality ~ age + sex + covid_
indicator + diabetes_indicator, data = data, family =
binomial())
summary(logistic_model)
```

Notice that we are again staying within the GLM framework but are using the binomial family to fit our model in both implementations.

In logistic regression, the coefficients are interpreted as the change in the log odds of the event occurring for a one-unit change in the predictor variable. A positive coefficient implies an increase in the likelihood of the event occurring, while a negative coefficient indicates a decrease. The regression coefficients are often converted to odds ratio for greater interpretability when modeling binary outcomes. Since the coefficients are modeled as log odds, we can exponentiate the log odds to obtain the odds ratio directly. For example, if the coefficient is 0.5, it suggests that the odds of the event happening increase by a factor of exp(0.5) (approximately 1.65) for each one-unit increase in the predictor variable.

Regression Assumptions

Now, we can't just go around running regression models willy-nilly. We must ensure that the data conditions are appropriate for the selected model. That is, we must check our assumptions. A common mnemonic for modeling a normal distribution is L.I.N.E., an acronym for (1) Linearity, (2) Independence of Errors, (3) Normality, and (4) Equal Variance.

Let's break these down a bit.

As discussed above, a fundamental assumption in linear regression is that the predictor variables have a *linear relationship* with the response. As the predictor value increases, we expect a proportional increase in the response variable by a factor of β. We can transform the predictor variables (e.g., using logs) on occasion so that the transformed predictor has a linear relationship with the response despite a non-linear relationship with the unadjusted predictor. The point here is that the relationship must be linear in the coefficients (despite these sneaky tricks to model non-linearity through transformations).

The *independence* of errors assumption states that a regression model's errors, also known as residuals, are independent. In other words, the error for one data point should not be related to the error for any other data point in the dataset. In healthcare, a typical scenario where this assumption can be violated is when evaluating patient outcomes whereby the same patient has multiple encounters with a care provider. Since the outcomes for the same patient are likely to be similar across encounters (e.g., high blood pressure), we can no longer state that the errors are independent in that the errors for a given patient across encounters are likely to be correlated. Ignoring the violation of the independence assumption in this context can lead to biased coefficients and incorrect statistical inferences.

To state the obvious, our third assumption is that when working with an OLS or GLM with a Gaussian distribution, the response variable being modeled must be *normal*. If the response distribution is not normal, our interpretation of the predictor variables may be misleading (or erroneous altogether), and the resulting predictions from our model can be misaligned. Of course, we've shown that many distributions do not conform to a normal distribution and can be modeled with GLMs using alternate distributions ("Poisson", "Negative Binomial", "Gamma", etc.). We can, therefore, restate this assumption as a "Distributional" assumption, meaning that the response distribution in the observed data must align with the distribution selected in the fitted model (e.g., GLM). LIDE doesn't have the same ring to it, so we'll stick with LINE for now.

Lastly is the assumption of *equal variance*, which states that the variance of the response variable should be constant across all levels of the predictor variables. In other words, the spread of the residuals should be roughly the same across the range of predictors. If we were to plot the residuals (i.e., the prediction minus our observed value) from a simple linear regression against the range of predictor variables, we should see equal variance across all values of the predictor. That is, we do not have a greater degree of error along some subset of the predictor values. Equal variance in fancy stats lingo, is referred to as homoscedasticity. If this assumption is violated, we see a fluting pattern of residuals called heteroscedasticity. Heteroscedasticity is generally characterized by an increasing degree of error as the value of the predictor increases.

Table 5.5 shows the applicability of various model assumptions to different types of regression models:

TABLE 5.5

Assumptions by Regression Model Type

Assumption	Linear Regression	Logistic Regression	Multinomial Regression	Poisson Regression	Negative Binomial Regression	Ordinal Regression
Linearity of Relationships	✓					
Independence of Errors	✓	✓	✓	✓	✓	✓
Normality of Errors	✓					
Equal Variance	✓	✓	✓	✓		
Categorical Dependent Variable		✓	✓			✓

While the LINE assumptions are the pillars of linear regression, some other assumptions about regression modeling are important to mention.

Like in linear regression, GLMs assume that there is no perfect multicollinearity among predictor variables. Perfect multicollinearity occurs when one predictor variable can be precisely predicted from the others. Adequate sample size is also essential, especially when dealing with rare events or fitting models with many predictors. Small sample sizes can lead to unstable coefficients and unreliable model results. We've used small samples for demonstration purposes in this book; however, in the real world, we would expect considerably more samples for valid analysis. Outliers or influential data points can affect the model's parameter estimates and goodness-of-fit measures. Identifying and influential data points is important in GLM analysis. We'll touch on this topic later, but suffice it to say that extreme data points can bias the model fit and result in suboptimal predictions. Lastly is the potential for overdispersion, which occurs when the response variable's variance is greater than expected from the chosen distribution. Underdispersion can also occur, which has the opposite characteristics. In the case of overdispersion, the negative binomial distribution can be employed in the GLM, which does not assume constant variance across the response distribution.

Measuring Model Fit

There's an old South Asian parable about a group of blind men encountering an elephant for the first time. Each person approaches the animal by touching it to understand what an elephant is. One person touches the flat elephant's ears, another touches its trunk-like legs, yet another touches its wall-like torso, and finally, another touches its narrow tail. Of course, the moral of the story is that each person has a different perspective of reality based on their unique experiences. Well, a fitted model is a bit like an elephant, and we, as blind analysts, must use various tests and visualizations to understand how a model is fit in multidimensional space. There are many quantitative metrics that provide insight into different aspects of model fit; however, relying on one metric exclusively can be misleading and result in an incomplete picture of performance.

If the model is designed solely to explore the relationship between predictors and a response (such as risk factors and an outcome), we might evaluate these metrics on the data used to fit the model—the study population or sample. However, if the goal is to use the model for out-of-sample predictions, it is typically assessed using training and testing (or derivation and validation) datasets. In this process, a portion of the data (e.g., 80%) is used to train the model, and the remaining 20% is reserved for testing, providing unseen data to evaluate the model's performance through a variety of metrics. More thorough methods, such as k-fold cross-validation, can also be applied so that all data can be used to fit and evaluate the model. This approach mitigates potential sampling error introduced by the testing dataset.

Assessing Model Fit in Healthcare Statistics: Linear, Logistic, and Poisson Regression

Let's review some standard techniques for measuring model fit. We'll simplify the discussion by considering model fit using linear, Poisson, and logistic regression.

Linear Regression Model Fit

I prefer to start with inspecting the results using a bivariate scatterplot. In this approach, the observed response variables are plotted on the x-axis, and the estimated values (i.e., our predictions) are plotted on the y-axis. I also prefer to add an alignment line with an intercept of 0 and a slope of 1 (Figure 5.2). An ideal model will show balanced error on both sides of the line, with constant variance across the observed response values without deviating in one direction. This visualization can also reveal outlier values that may affect model fit.

The mean squared error (MSE) is another helpful metric, especially when incremental improvements to model fit are difficult to detect visually (or when we report model fit in presentations, white papers, and publications). MSE is the mean of the squared residuals (i.e., the differences between our predictions and observed values).

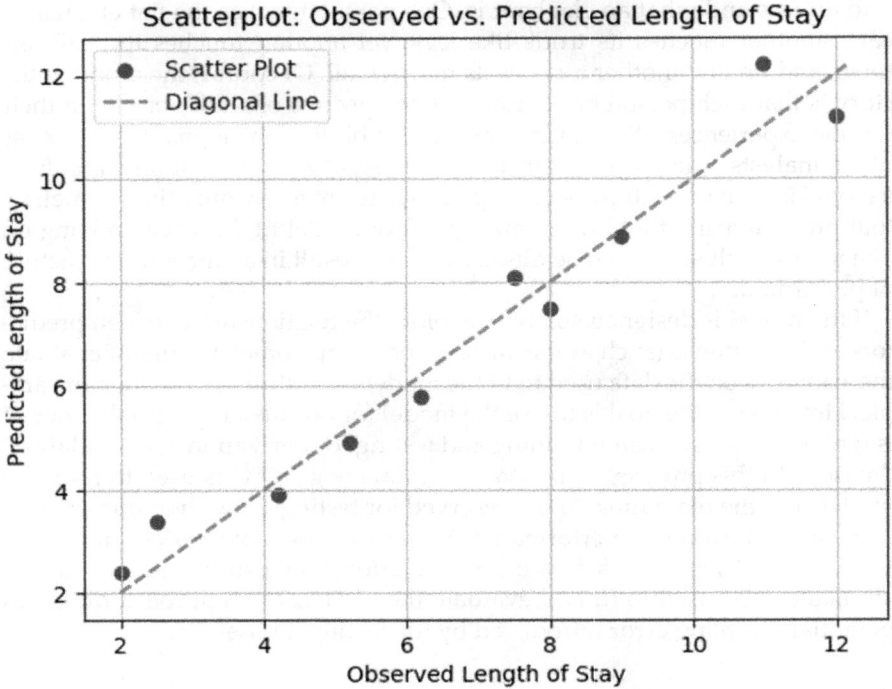

FIGURE 5.2
Visualization of an example of OLS regression fit.

R-squared and Pearson's correlation coefficient are also useful metrics that quantify the percentage of variation in the response by the model predictors. Still, we would not want to rely on these metrics exclusively. It is quite possible for a model to have a high R-square value while exhibiting a sub-optimal fit. For example, a slight nonlinear relationship between the predicted and observed values may exist despite a high R-square value. Overall, the model may be performing satisfactorily, but a greater degree of error might exist on the extremes of the response distribution.

Collectively evaluating the model through a combination of these techniques will, like the blind men, prove the most complete picture of our model.

Logistic Regression Model Fit

With logistic regression, the outcome variable is binary. While we can attempt to plot the residuals as we did with linear regression, a more interpretable visualization is the box plot. In this visualization, separate box and whisker plots for observed positive and negative cases (i.e., cases with the outcome and cases without) are plotted against the probabilities produced from the logistic regression model. Using this approach, we assess the range of values for each outcome (positive and negative), aiming to create greater separation between the two distributions. A logistic regression that perfectly discriminates between positive and negative cases (assuming a probability threshold value) will exhibit no overlap in the distributions (represented through the box and whiskers). Figure 5.3 shows the boxplot comparing estimated probability distribution between true cases of readmissions and non-readmissions.

A confusion matrix, as shown in Table 5.6, is also an incredibly helpful tool to quantify different types of model error. Perhaps we're predicting CAUTIs (catheter-associated urinary tract infections) for inpatients as part of a real-time alerting tool. Our model might predict high CAUTI risk on a patient's age, catheter days, and other infections. There are times

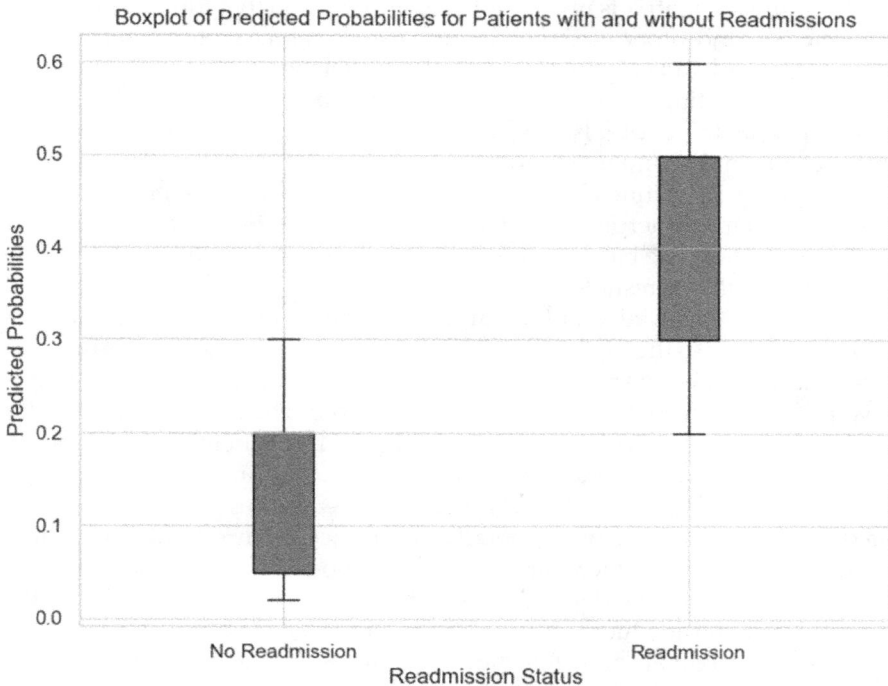

FIGURE 5.3
Boxplot comparing the predicted probability distributions between observed readmitted and non-readmitted cases.

TABLE 5.6

A Confusion Matrix Comparing Predictions Versus Reality

		Reality	
		Yes	**No**
Prediction	**Yes**	True Positive	False Positive (Type I Error)
	No	False Negative (Type II Error)	True Negative

when we will predict high CAUTI risk when no CAUTI develops. This scenario would be considered a false positive. It is a false alarm. Another scenario would be the occurrence of CAUTI when our model predicts low CAUTI risk. This scenario would be considered a false negative. Other scenarios could be that we predict low CAUTI risk and no CAUTI occurs (a true negative), or we predict high CAUTI risk, and CAUTI does happen (a true positive).

The confusion matrix is my favorite communication tool for logistic regression models and other classification models for clinical stakeholders. It is straightforward and easy to explain. If the model were to be implemented in a production setting, everyone would have an upfront understanding of the types (false positives or false negatives) and respective expected frequencies of the errors in the employed model.

The receiver operating characteristic (ROC) curve, as shown in Figure 5.4, is another helpful metric in evaluating models with binary outcomes. It is designed to show the balance of the true positive rate and false positive rate across probability thresholds.

The ideal model using an ROC curve would show the bend of the curve as close as possible to the top left corner—with 100% true positives and 0% false positives. A related metric is the area under the curve (AUC) metric, which quantifies the percentage of data under the curve. The AUC would be 1 (or 100%) in our perfect scenario discussed above. The benefit of this metric is that it is a threshold-less method of evaluating model fit.

If we use the logistic regression model to measure associations between predictors and response, we generally do not need a threshold value—that is, the probability at which we will predict a positive case. However, if we want to deploy our model and make predictions, we must decide on the probability value at which we identify a positive case. In our CAUTI alerting example, we might alert the infection preventionist when a high CAUTI risk is detected.

How do we pick a probability threshold? One method would be using a metric that balances true and false positives. A probability threshold that is

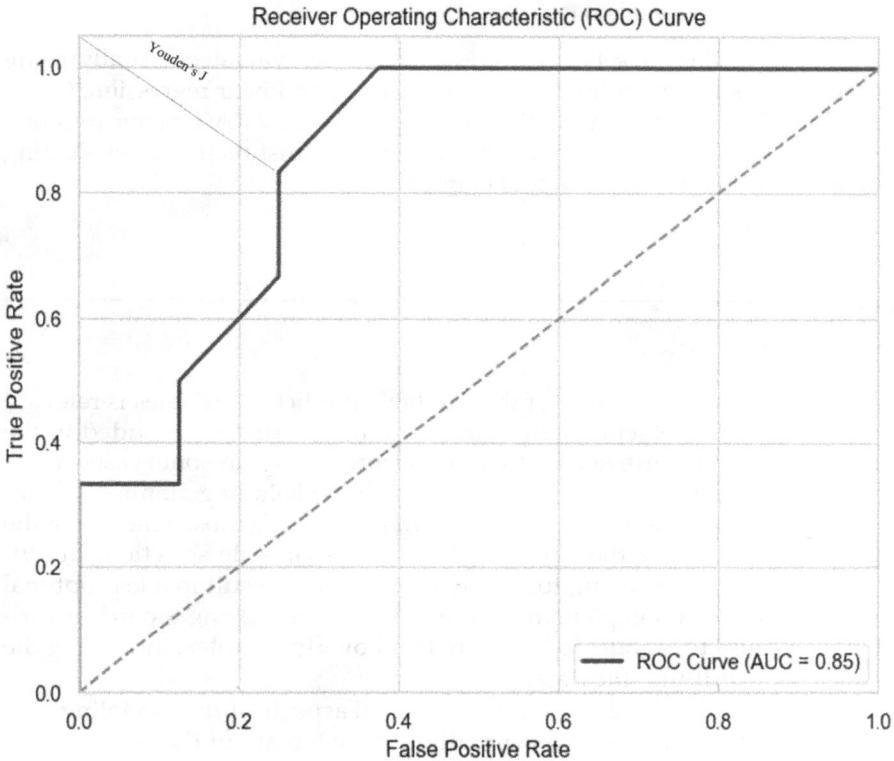

FIGURE 5.4
Example Receiving Operating Characteristic (ROC) Curve with Youden's J Statistic as an optimal probability threshold.

too high will improve the accuracy of the predictions we make but might increase our false negatives. A low probability threshold might increase our false positive rate (due to making predictions with lower probabilities). Youden's J statistic is a threshold value that balances true positives with false positives by identifying the point on the ROC curve closest to the top left corner (the theoretical point of perfect fit). It is essentially the point of the curve that minimizes the Euclidean distance to the perfect point.

An analogous measure to MSE for logistic regression is deviance. While a bit less interpretable, it is a valid relative measure to assess model fit, especially when experimenting with alternative models and evaluating the utility of additional predictors.

Poisson Regression Model Fit

Poisson regression, like linear regression, can be evaluated visually using scatterplots as described in the previous section on linear regression. Given that Logistic regression and Poisson regression are GLMs using different distributions, the deviance metric can also be a robust metric for evaluating incremental changes to the model to improve fit.

Variable Selection

In many cases, only a subset of the available predictor variables is relevant to our business problem. Being selective about predictors included in the model can provide greater focus and interpretability. In some cases, there may be hundreds or thousands (especially in the field of genomics) of candidate predictors that we must sift through to identify those relevant to the model. This is where the game is played with variable selection. In outcomes modeling, removing too many variables can result in a less optimal model, as important explanatory information is lost. Using too many variables can cause the model to be bloated and overly complex, increasing the chances of overfitting the data.

I believe that this is one of the most critical aspects of the modeling process. Newcomers to the field generally get excited about the range of statistical models themselves and all the clever dials (hyperparameters) that can be tuned to improve model fit. Far more important than fine-tuning the technical aspects of the model is ensuring that the variables included are appropriate for the research question. Carefully curating a set of predictors will result in a more credible model that can be defended when presenting to clinical stakeholders. While we need to use data-driven strategies for selecting variables in many instances, there should always be a balance between domain knowledge and the technical process used to select variables.

In this section, we'll discuss some strategies for selecting variables and their benefits and drawbacks.

Data-Driven Variable Selection

Stepwise variable selection is usually the first strategy suggested when attempting to limit the number of predictor variables in a model. This process involves either incrementally adding variables (forward selection) or incrementally removing variables (backward selection) and assessing model fit with each iteration to determine if the evaluated variable should be included (or excluded). An even more thorough approach is to use a combination of forward and backward selection. In this process, performance metrics such as the *Akaike information criterion (AIC)* or the more conservative *Bayesian Information Criterion (BIC)*, are used to balance model complexity with model fit. Only variables that help materially explain the outcome are retained in the model in this process. In this scenario, highly correlated variables will likely be excluded from the stepwise process.

Another challenge with stepwise models is that they can be computationally intensive, as a model is fit for each iteration in the forward and backward stepwise process. While stepwise modeling is generally the most common data-driven method for variable selection, it can also be dangerous, especially when used to predict health outcomes.

> Here's an example: let us say we are evaluating a broad set of chronic conditions to understand their association with readmission occurrences in the med/surg setting. Our stepwise model considers both Type II diabetes and hypertension, among many other variables. In the stepwise process, it is determined that the Type 2 diabetes predictor contributes significantly to the model, and hypertension evaluated in another iteration in the stepwise process is excluded for not adding materially to the model fit beyond the information captured in the Type II diabetes variable.

While the model fit might be improved (complexity being considered), we could end up with a model that accounts for the mortality risk for patients with hypertension but not Type II diabetes. No additional risk is detected for the hypertension patient because we've excluded that variable from the model.

Another comon approach for variable selection is through regression models that penalize coefficients from being too extreme to the point that some coefficients are either reduced to zero or have minimal influence on the model. This family of "penalized regression" includes models such as Lasso and Ridge regression. These, too, can result in similar challenges (as correlated variables may be excluded (or minimized); however, they are quite efficient at optimizing as the model is only fit once, and the beta coefficients are iteratively reduced through a secondary process. We'll talk more about these in the section on highly dimensional data (as they are used as a preliminary variable selection technique and standalone models on their own).

Manual Curation

There is danger in the mindset of just letting the algorithm figure out the right variables (an all-too-common approach in many organizations). An approach at the other extreme is the manual selection of predictors based on subject matter expertise. This approach produces models that are well-grounded in domain knowledge and easy to defend. The drawback of this method is that we might overlook essential predictors. Human subject matter experts will provide important information but often cannot readily catalog all potential risk factors from memory (or even through a review of the academic literature). Data-driven methods are great at bringing important candidate variables to the table for consideration that may not be on top of mind to subject matter experts.

A Hybrid Approach

Generally, the preferred approach is a hybrid of the data-driven assessment of the data and the manual curation of variables to refine the candidate set of predictors further. One way to go about a hybrid approach would be to fit univariate models for each potential predictor. We could, for example, iterate over a set of comorbidities for conditions present on admission to surface candidate variables that have a statistically significant association with the outcome of interest. This process can serve as an initial filter so the subject matter experts can further reduce the predictors to those that make clinical sense.

One might ask, why not just run a multiple regression model to see which variables are significant? Is the univariate approach necessary? The difficulty is the potential correlation of variables. Correlated variables can often result in sign changes of the coefficients (a change from positive to negative or vice versa). As a result, blindly throwing all variables into a model might muddy the waters.

Once a subject matter expert reviews a set of statistically significant variables (from the univariate model), we have a base set of validated candidate variables that may be considered in the final stages of modeling. In my opinion, a hybrid approach, when possible, results in a model that is clinically valid but informed by known associations in the data.

TLDR: A combination of domain knowledge and data-driven methods should be considered for variable selection Figure 5.5.

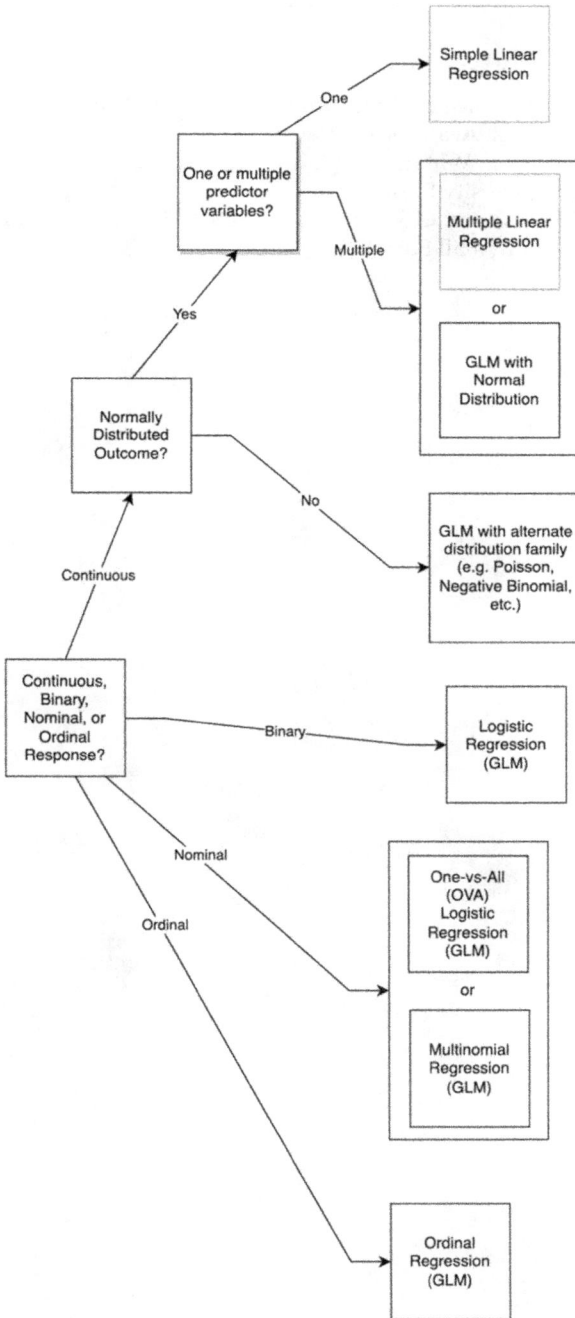

FIGURE 5.5
Workflow for choosing an appropriate regression model.

Additional Resources

James, G., Witten, D., Hastie, T., & Tibshirani, R. (2021). *Introduction to Statistical Learning*. Springer. Available online: https://www.statlearning.com

Gelman, A., Hill, J., & Vehtari, A. (2020). *Regression and Other Stories* (1st ed.). Cambridge University Press.

Kutner, M. H., Nachtsheim, C. J., & Neter, J. (2004). *Applied Linear Statistical Models* (5th ed.). McGraw-Hill Education.

6

Advanced Regression Modeling

As statisticians, data scientists, and researchers, we regularly encounter new data scenarios, and on occasion, basic methods, such as linear, Poisson, and logistic regression, will be insufficient.

In this section, we will discuss a broader range of models and techniques that are often excluded from a beginner's guide. While it is not possible to provide an exhaustive review of these methods, I do think it's vital that the reader be aware of them so that they may be pursued further when encountering these more challenging scenarios. In my experience, these are the models that newcomers often lack knowledge of, causing them to jump too quickly to ML-based approaches.

The content in this section is problem-based, and in some cases, multiple options are provided to address specific data scenarios.

This will be a bit of a speed dating session to see if a model might be a good fit for your data problem. Like any relationship, you might find a good match, but I encourage you to get to know these models to understand their unique quirks before fully committing. Additional resources are provided at the end of this chapter, along with some recommended readings. Table 6.1 further provides an overview of the data scenarios analysts will likely encounter that might lead them to abandon regression methods. With each data scenario, a proposed regression variant is suggested as an intermediate step before making the leap to a fully blown ML approach.

Non-linearity

Earlier in this chapter, I mentioned that generalized additive models (GAMs) are my secret weapon when presented with challenges of non-linearity. Here's a real-world example. In evaluating the risk of maternal complications, both pediatric pregnancies (younger mothers) and geriatric pregnancies (older mothers) have an increased risk of eclampsia—a life-threatening complication of pregnancy characterized by sudden development of seizures.

TABLE 6.1

Modeling Options for Common Data Scenarios

Problem	Options
Non-linear relationship between response and predictor	Option 1: Transformations of response and/or predictors (log, quadratic, cubic transformations) Option 2: GAMs (using spline functions)
Data is highly correlated	Option 1: Stepwise Modeling Option 2: Penalized Regression (Lasso/Ridge) Option 3: Regression with Principal Components (my preference)
Multiple response variables	Option 1: Stratification: One vs. All (OVA) Option 2: Mutinomial/Multivariate Regression (depending on outcome type)
Multiple levels of data	Option 1: Mixed-effect/hierarchical models
Response variable has lots of zeros	Option 1: Zero-inflated regression
Response is ordinal	Option 1: Ordinal regression
Outcome is dependent on exposure/observation time	Option 1: Rate regression
Complex interaction among predictors	1. Manual curation of interaction terms (my preference when possible) 2. Penalized regression (Lasso Ridge) 3. Consider alternative models (e.g., tree-based models)

Regression coefficients are suitable for identifying linear relationships, so a linear coefficient would be acceptable if risk increases proportionately with age. In the case of eclampsia, we can observe a parabola-shaped risk curve, whereby younger and older patients are at greater risk for eclampsia, with a lower-risk population in the middle of the age range.

With non-linear relationships, we could consider transforming the predictor variable itself. For example, we might experiment with log, quadratic, or cubic transformations to improve the linear fit. We could also consider binning the data so that each segment is its own categorical variable. However, there is a point at which complex non-linear relationships cannot easily be modeled through simple transformations of the predictors. At that point, we must seek out more robust methods.

Enter GAMs. The beauty of a GAM is that complex nonlinear relationships between each predictor variable and response using spline functions—which are piecewise-defined polynomial functions designed to model nonlinear relationships. *There you go again, Michael, with your fancy word soup.* I'm sorry. Let me explain.

A spline function is a mathematical function that shows continuous change over the range of predictor variables. The optimization process in a GAM will divide the predictor variable into segments (smaller ranges) and fit a relatively simple polynomial equation to each segment. The connection points between segments (i.e., "knots") are further constrained to be continuous, ensuring smooth transitions between the knots. This construction allows splines to capture complex, non-linear patterns in data while maintaining smoothness. Note that splines are generally the preferred smoothing function, but other functions can be employed.

In short, we can use a GAM when a non-linear relationship between our predictor and response variable cannot be resolved through simple transformations to our predictor variables. I prefer to use spline functions for patient age for example, as patient risk is naturally non-linear. Depending on the disease group being evaluated, the risk of an outcome can vary considerably across age ranges, as the risk of mortality between ages 20 and 30 is much different than the change in risk between ages 70 and 80, despite both being a ten-year increase in age. A spine function will naturally account for the varying risk across age groups.

For demonstration, it is easy to conceptualize a GAM model for a continuous response. It should be noted that GAMs, like GLMs, can also be used to model other data distributions in the exponential family of distributions (e.g., binomial, Poisson, gamma).

$$\text{Length of Stay} = \text{Intercept} + f(Age) + \varepsilon$$

Or more generally

$$Y = \alpha + f(X) + \varepsilon$$

where

$f(Age)$ represents a smooth function of age to capture non-linear between age and LOS.

Let's look at an example implementation in Python.

```
import pandas as pd
from pygam import LinearGAM, s
import matplotlib.pyplot as plt
import numpy as np

data = {
    'Age': [25, 30, 40, 50, 60, 35, 45, 55, 65, 75, 25,
30, 40, 50, 60, 35, 45, 55, 65, 75],
    'Length_of_Stay': [1, 1, 19, 34, 67, 10, 20, 42, 91,
143, 8, 1, 13, 34, 66, 4, 15, 60, 90, 144]
}

df = pd.DataFrame(data)
gam = LinearGAM(s(0), verbose=True).fit(df[['Age']],
np.log(df['Length_of_Stay']))
print(gam.summary())
intercept_value = gam.predict(np.array([[0]]))  # Provide
a data point with Age set to 0
print("Intercept Value:", intercept_value[0])
```

```
XX = gam.generate_X_grid(term=0)
pdep, confi = gam.partial_dependence(term=0, X=XX,
width=0.95)

plt.figure()
plt.plot(XX, pdep)
plt.fill_between(XX[:, 0], confi[:, 0], confi[:, 1],
alpha=0.3)
plt.title("Partial Dependence Plot for Age")
plt.xlabel("Age")
plt.ylabel("Partial Dependence")
plt.xlim(25, 75)  # Limit the x-axis to the age range of
25 to 75
plt.show()
```

Figure 6.1 shows the "partial dependence" plot of the age predictor variable, modeled as a spline function in our GAM against length of stay (log-transformed) as our response variable.

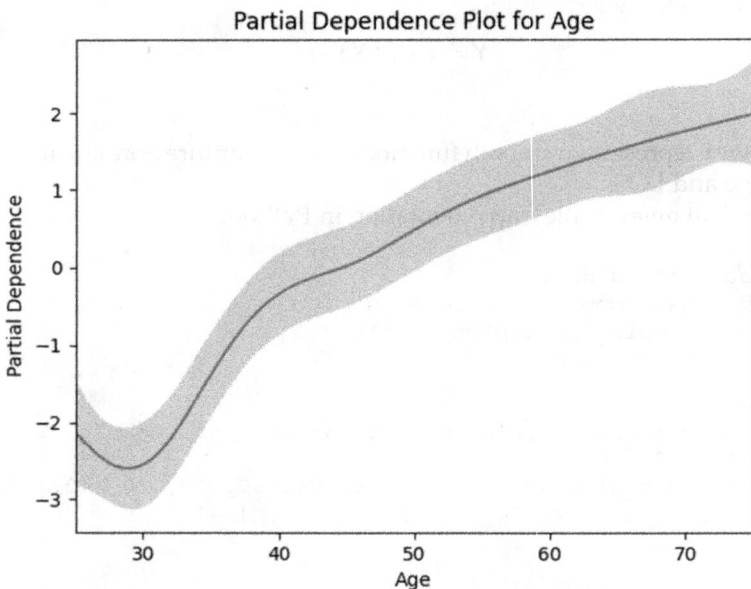

FIGURE 6.1
Partial dependence plot for the age predictor variable used in a GAM.

The plot's primary curve demonstrates the outcome variable's partial dependence on the selected feature. It shows how the predicted outcome changes as the predictor "Age" increases. Notice that the log length of stay risk increases nonlinearly with age.

Also, notice the shaded areas around the main curve representing confidence intervals. These intervals depict the model's uncertainty about its predictions. Wider intervals indicate greater uncertainty about the associations at that range of the predictor. It is common to see the error bands flute at the two ends of the range of predictor values as fewer data points generally exist at the edges, resulting in more uncertainty.

We can accomplish the same results using the mgcv in R to fit the GAM model

```
library(mgcv)

data <- data.frame(
  Age = c(25, 30, 40, 50, 60, 35, 45, 55, 65, 75, 25, 30,
40, 50, 60, 35, 45, 55, 65, 75),
  Length_of_Stay = c(1, 1, 19, 34, 67, 10, 20, 42, 91,
143, 8, 1, 13, 34, 66, 4, 15, 60, 90, 144)
)

gam_model <- gam(log(Length_of_Stay) ~ s(Age), data =
data, method = "REML")

summary(gam_model)

intercept_value <- predict(gam_model, newdata = data.
frame(Age = 0))
print(paste("Intercept Value:", intercept_value))

age_grid <- seq(25, 75, length.out = 100)
partial_dep <- predict(gam_model, newdata = data.
frame(Age = age_grid), type = "link")

plot(age_grid, partial_dep, type = "l", col = "blue", lwd
= 2,
     xlab = "Age", ylab = "Partial Dependence",
     main = "Partial Dependence Plot for Age")
```

Highly Correlated Variables (Multicollinearity)

One of the most vexing aspects of modeling clinical data is the correlation between a patient's diagnoses and procedures. Often, one comorbidity is part of the causal pathway of another (e.g., hypertension and Type II Diabetes). Additionally, procedures and other services are conditional on other diagnoses (e.g., amputation of the toes for Type II Diabetics). As such, it makes sense that diagnoses and procedures are highly correlated.

Highly correlated variables or *multicollinearity* can result in erroneous sign changes in the coefficients, further inflating their standard error. We touched on this topic in the variable selection section of this chapter. Still, given the disastrous effects of highly correlated variables on interpreting predictor and response associations, it is worth dedicating more time to it.

Building a correlation matrix showing the degree to which the predictor variables are correlated (and the direction of that correlation) can be helpful in the data exploration process. I see this as a critical step in the modeling process; however, it is not sufficient on its own (Figure 6.2).

Sometimes, one variable may not be directly correlated with other predictor variables, but it is redundant through the linear combination of other variables. That is, some predictor variables can be approximated through the combined information of other predictor variables. This, too, can cause similar issues with the interpretation of model coefficients.

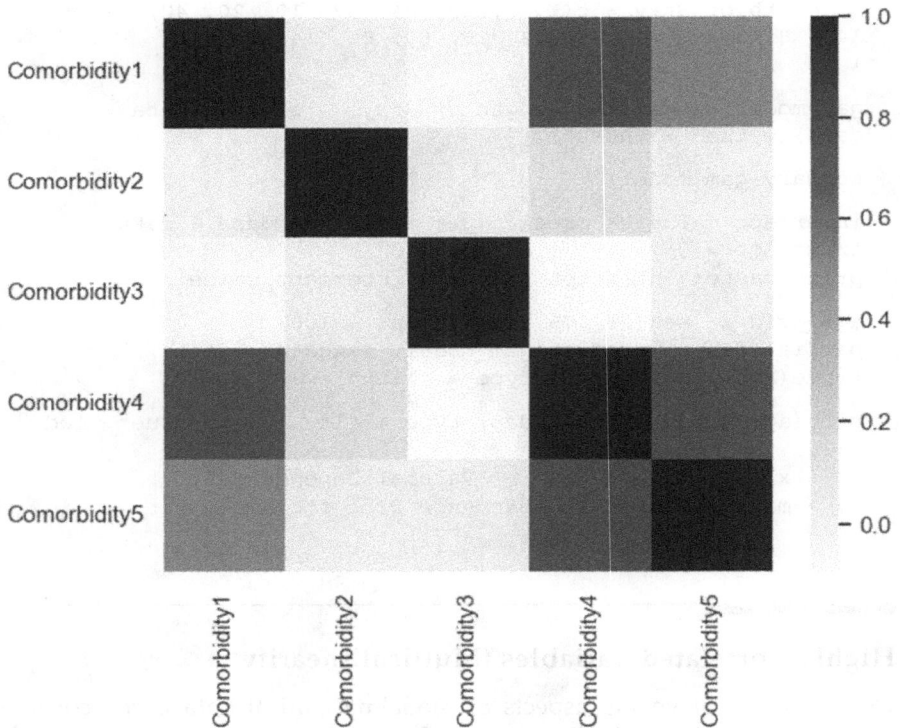

FIGURE 6.2
Correlation plot showing correlation among predictor variables.

Variance Inflation Factors

The variance inflation factor (or VIF) is a common technique for identifying such variables. The VIF helps us understand how much the accuracy of our regression model might be affected by multicollinearity. It quantifies how much the variance is inflated in our model coefficients.

If we have a model with several correlated predictors, the VIF, for example, "BMI", is calculated by regressing each predictor variable on the other predictor variables and measuring the increase in its variance (e.g., "weight" and "height"). The larger the VIF, the more its variance is inflated due to its correlation with other predictors.

Let's look at an example calculation of the VIF in Python using a model where a complication is being predicted from a set of comorbidities.

```
import pandas as pd
import numpy as np
from statsmodels.stats.outliers_influence import
variance_inflation_factor
from statsmodels.tools.tools import add_constant
from sklearn.linear_model import LogisticRegression

np.random.seed(123)

df = pd.DataFrame({
    'Comorbidity1': np.random.rand(100),
    'Comorbidity2': np.random.rand(100) + 0.1,
    'Comorbidity3': np.random.rand(100) + 0.05,
    'Comorbidity4': np.random.rand(100) + 0.09,
    'Comorbidity5': np.random.rand(100) + 0.7,
    'Complication': np.random.choice([0, 1], size=100)
})

X = add_constant(df[['Comorbidity1', 'Comorbidity2',
'Comorbidity3', 'Comorbidity4', 'Comorbidity5']])
y = df['Complication']

vif_results = pd.DataFrame()
vif_results['Variable'] = X.columns
vif_results['VIF'] = [variance_inflation_factor(X.values,
i) for i in range(X.shape[1])]

print("VIF results:\n", vif_results)
```

In R, we can use the `vif` function from the car package to accomplish the same results:

```
library(car)
set.seed(123)
df <- data.frame(
  Comorbidity1 = runif(100),
  Comorbidity2 = runif(100) + 0.1,
  Comorbidity3 = runif(100) + 0.05,
  Comorbidity4 = runif(100) + 0.09,
  Comorbidity5 = runif(100) + 0.7,
  Complication = sample(c(0, 1), 100, replace = TRUE)
)

lm_model <- lm(Complication ~ Comorbidity1 + Comorbidity2
+ Comorbidity3 + Comorbidity4 + Comorbidity5, data = df)

vif_results <- vif(lm_model)

print(vif_results)
```

To interpret VIF values, a VIF of 1 means that there's no correlation between the evaluated predictor and the other predictors, so the variance is not inflated. Generally, VIFs exceeding 4 suggest a need for investigation, and VIFs over 10 indicate serious multicollinearity that should be addressed in your model.

When we encounter scenarios where variables contain duplicative information, we can surgically correct them. For example, we might group two similar variables into a broader indicator or category so that neither is excluded. We could also create an interaction term (the product of the two variables) so that the cooccurrence of those variables is controlled for in the modeling process (more on this later).

Principal Component Analysis in Regression

A few years ago, I collaborated with a team of statisticians, researchers, clinicians, and public health practitioners to better understand the association between social drivers of health (SDoHs) and clinical outcomes across certain disease groups. Our goal was to capture multiple aspects of SDoH, but we were concerned about the duplicative information in many of the variables in the dataset. Variables related to home value, access to transportation, income, disability, and uninsured status generally correlate but contain unique information that might explain a patient's health status. Our goal was to look across the variables to identify the unique aspects of SDoH risk across those variables. This is precisely the type of problem that principal component analysis (PCA) is designed to address. It is useful when we have a dataset comprising correlated variables, especially when it is highly dimensional (e.g., many predictors).

The finesse of PCA is that we can extract unique aspects of the data across variables. If you talk to statisticians about PCA, they might describe this process as mapping variables to lower-dimensional space. The result with PCA is a set of *principal components*—each capturing a unique uncorrelated aspect of the data. For the SDoH example, the first principal component might capture aspects of wealth (that are captured across variables like income, home value, and uninsured status). Another principal component might capture aspects of disability, while another might capture aspects of rurality. Note that it is not always clear what aspect of the data is being captured (but there are tricks we can use to help make principal components more explainable).

The derived principal components can be used in a compressed (or lower-dimensional) form of a larger set of variables to simplify the algorithm and mitigate data redundancy issues. Structurally, PCA generates principal components that do not correlate with each other. We can, in turn, use these principal components as predictor variables in the regression (rather than the raw predictor variables from which they are derived).

$$Y = \alpha + \beta_1 PC_1 + \ldots + \beta_n PC_n$$

With PCA, we can have our cake and eat it, too—that is, we can use all the variables without concern for multicollinearity, and we are not forced to exclude variables that include potentially helpful information, as is the case with stepwise variable selection and penalized regression.

PCA is an *unsupervised* method that derives the principal components without a response variable. We are simply extracting the unique aspects of the data that are most dominant across all variables. Each principal component explains some degree of variation in the data, so the cumulative variance explained by all principal components would be 100%. It is important to select a subset of the principal components that capture most, but not all, of the variation in the data.

A "scree plot" is a valuable tool for visualizing the percent of variation explained by each principal component. With highly correlated data, the first few principal components should explain a larger share of the total variance. With data that has minimal correlation, we should see less disparity between the variation explained by the principal components.

Different strategies exist for selecting the ideal number of principal components. One common approach is to take all the principal components necessary to explain 80% of the variation in the data. This approach can be challenging, depending on how imbalanced the variation explained across the principal components is. Another method, which is a bit of an art form (but perfectly valid), is to identify the inflection point where we see a precipitous drop in the variation explained in the scree plot.

Let's look at a "scree plot" as part of this process.

In this example (Figure 6.3), the first two components explain most of the variation in the data, so we might choose this limited set of principal components to use as predictors in our final model.

PCA is sensitive to the magnitude and skew in the data, so an important preprocessing step is to center and scale the data (typically with z-score scaling). Otherwise, a variable like income will overpower other variables, such as food insecurity, simply due to magnitude. Another limitation is that PCA performs best with continuous variables (although a sprinkling of binary variables will not be too disruptive). If the dataset used for the analysis is all (or primarily) binary, there are variants of PCA better suited for those datasets.

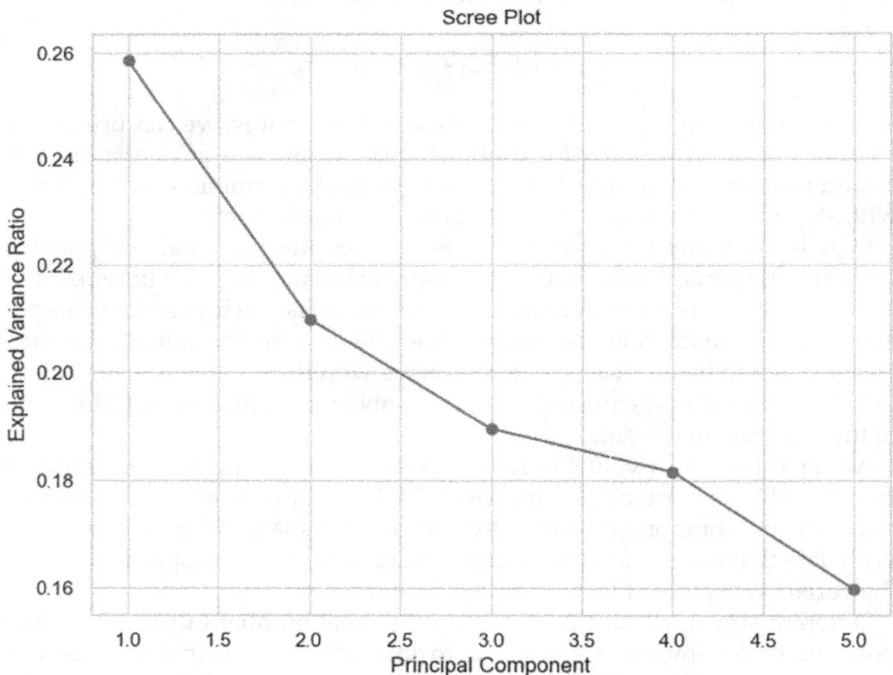

FIGURE 6.3
Scree plot from PCA model showing the percentage of variance explained with each principal component.

Let's now look at a more complete picture of how PCA can be used in conjunction with regression to overcome challenges with multicollinearity. In this problem, we have a response variable (30-day readmission) with a set of correlated SDoH variables (education, income, housing, food insecurity, transportation, and social support).

Python

```python
import pandas as pd
import numpy as np
import statsmodels.api as sm
from sklearn.decomposition import PCA
from sklearn.preprocessing import StandardScaler

data = {
    'Education': [12, 14, 10, 16, 8, 12, 14, 13, 15, 11,
12, 14, 10, 16, 8, 12, 14, 13, 15, 11],
    'Income': [35000, 42000, 30000, 52000, 25000, 33000,
41000, 39000, 48000, 29000, 35000, 42000, 30000, 52000,
25000, 33000, 41000, 39000, 48000, 29000],
    'Employment': [1, 0, 1, 1, 0, 1, 0, 1, 1, 0, 1, 0, 1,
1, 0, 1, 0, 1, 1, 0],
    'Housing': [1, 1, 0, 1, 0, 1, 0, 1, 1, 0, 1, 1, 0, 1,
0, 1, 0, 1, 1, 0],
    'FoodSecurity': [3, 2, 1, 3, 1, 2, 1, 3, 3, 1, 3, 2,
1, 3, 1, 2, 1, 3, 3, 1],
    'Transportation': [1, 0, 1, 1, 0, 1, 0, 1, 1, 0, 1,
0, 1, 1, 0, 1, 0, 1, 1, 0],
    'SocialSupport': [4, 3, 3, 5, 2, 4, 3, 5, 5, 2, 4, 3,
3, 5, 2, 4, 3, 5, 5, 2],
    'CommunitySafety': [3, 2, 2, 4, 1, 3, 2, 4, 4, 1, 3,
2, 2, 4, 1, 3, 2, 4, 4, 1],
    'AccessToHealthcare': [1, 0, 1, 1, 0, 1, 0, 1, 1, 0,
1, 0, 1, 1, 0, 1, 0, 1, 1, 0],
    'AirQuality': [2, 3, 2, 3, 1, 2, 3, 2, 2, 1, 2, 3, 2,
3, 1, 2, 3, 2, 2, 1],
    '30DayReadmission': [1, 0, 1, 1, 0, 1, 0, 1, 1, 0, 1,
0, 1, 1, 0, 1, 0, 1, 0, 1],
}

df = pd.DataFrame(data)

X = df.drop('30DayReadmission', axis=1)
y = df['30DayReadmission']

scaler = StandardScaler()
X_scaled = scaler.fit_transform(X)
```

```
pca = PCA(n_components=2)
principal_components = pca.fit_transform(X_scaled)

pca_df = pd.DataFrame(data=principal_components,
columns=['PC1', 'PC2'])

pca_df['30DayReadmission'] = y

X_pca = sm.add_constant(pca_df[['PC1', 'PC2']])
model = sm.Logit(y, X_pca)
result = model.fit()

print(result.summary())
```

R

```
library(stats)
library(caret)

set.seed(123)

df <- data.frame(
  Education = c(12, 14, 10, 16, 8, 12, 14, 13, 15, 11,
12, 14, 10, 16, 8, 12, 14, 13, 15, 11),
  Income = c(35000, 42000, 30000, 52000, 25000, 33000,
41000, 39000, 48000, 29000, 35000, 42000, 30000, 52000,
25000, 33000, 41000, 39000, 48000, 29000),
  Employment = c(1, 0, 1, 1, 0, 1, 0, 1, 1, 0, 1, 0, 1,
1, 0, 1, 0, 1, 1, 0),
  Housing = c(1, 1, 0, 1, 0, 1, 0, 1, 1, 0, 1, 1, 0, 1,
0, 1, 0, 1, 1, 0),
  FoodSecurity = c(3, 2, 1, 3, 1, 2, 1, 3, 3, 1, 3, 2, 1,
3, 1, 2, 1, 3, 3, 1),
  Transportation = c(1, 0, 1, 1, 0, 1, 0, 1, 1, 0, 1, 0,
1, 1, 0, 1, 0, 1, 1, 0),
  SocialSupport = c(4, 3, 3, 5, 2, 4, 3, 5, 5, 2, 4, 3,
3, 5, 2, 4, 3, 5, 5, 2),
  CommunitySafety = c(3, 2, 2, 4, 1, 3, 2, 4, 4, 1, 3, 2,
2, 4, 1, 3, 2, 4, 4, 1),
  AccessToHealthcare = c(1, 0, 1, 1, 0, 1, 0, 1, 1, 0, 1,
0, 1, 1, 0, 1, 0, 1, 1, 0),
  AirQuality = c(2, 3, 2, 3, 1, 2, 3, 2, 2, 1, 2, 3, 2,
3, 1, 2, 3, 2, 2, 1),
  ThirtyDayReadmission = c(1, 0, 1, 1, 0, 1, 0, 1, 1, 0,
1, 0, 1, 1, 0, 1, 0, 1, 0, 1)
)
X <- df[, -which(names(df) == "ThirtyDayReadmission")]
y <- df$ThirtyDayReadmission
```

```
X_scaled <- scale(X)

pca_result <- prcomp(X_scaled, center = TRUE, scale. =
TRUE)
principal_components <- pca_result$x[, 1:2]  # Select the
first two principal components

pca_df <- data.frame(PC1 = principal_components[, 1], PC2
= principal_components[, 2])
pca_df$ThirtyDayReadmission <- y

model <- glm(ThirtyDayReadmission ~ PC1 + PC2, data =
pca_df, family = binomial)

summary(model)
```

In this case, PCA is a preprocessing step that compresses this set of correlated variables before using them in a logistic regression (i.e., a GLM with a binomial distribution).

But Mike, how can I explain a principal component to a clinician stakeholder? That doesn't seem very explainable to me. We are admittedly sacrificing some interpretability to have more complete and useful data with PCA. That said, some tricks can help us in these conversations.

My favorite method when explaining regression models that use PCA is to build a correlation matrix between the principal components and the original predictor variables. Let's explain this by way of example.

We can see in the mock data provided in Figure 6.4 that the first principal component is correlated with the most variables (which is the expected behavior with PCA). It is the component that is explaining the most dominant aspect of the data set. Notice that as we move to the second principal component, it is generally correlated with different predictor variables than the first components. Remember, PCA is designed to capture unique uncorrelated (i.e., orthogonal) aspects of variation in the data. With each principal component, we can see less variation being explained by the additional components (which aligns nicely with our scree plot).

I have found that this type of visualization is helpful in that it clearly shows which variables are correlated with each principal component. In many cases, the cluster of variables associated with a principal component can be given an intuitive name (e.g., "aspects of poverty", or "aspects of rurality) to help the consumer understand the how the principal component variables play a part subsequent fitted model.

When using PCA in a regression model, we can interpret the coefficients in the same way. We can say for example that there is a statistically

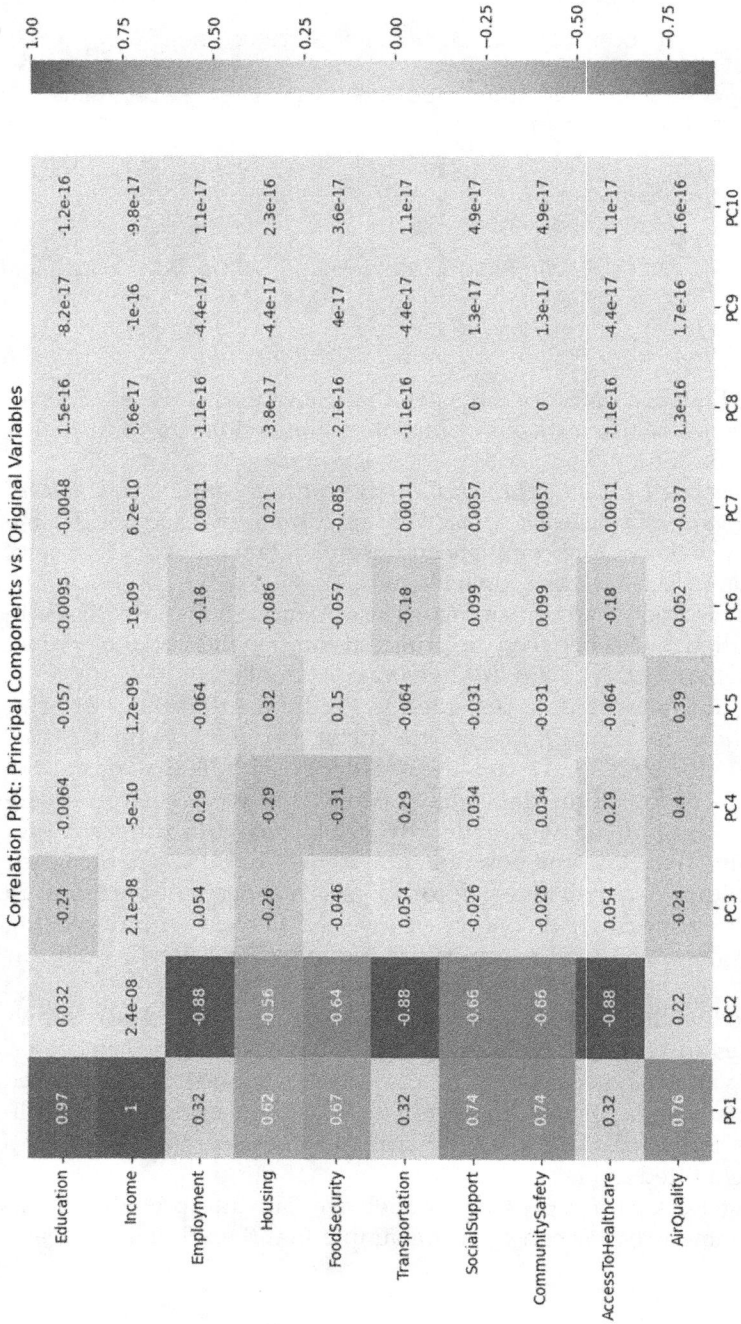

FIGURE 6.4
Correlation between the raw predictor variables and their derived principal components.

significant association between *aspects of poverty* and mortality. We might even include a set of raw variables (such as age, sex, and disease group) as predictors along with the SDoH principal components to understand the associations between SDoH principal components, after controlling for patient clinical and demographic characteristics. That is, we have the option to compress certain domains of data that are high-dimensional in nature and use them along with other variables outside of the PCA modeling.

Multiple Response Variables

The models discussed at the beginning of this chapter involved one response variable; however, there are times when the research question considers the possibility of multiple outcomes. As discussed in Chapter 2, there is the potential for a host of complications within the inpatient setting, including CMS Hospital Acquired Conditions (HACs), NHSN HAIs, and AHRQ Patient Safety Indicators (PSIs). Warning: Acronym overload! See Chapter 2 if these didn't make any sense. In our research question, perhaps we want to know the probabilities associated with each complication, conditional on a set of patient characteristics. Let's consider a few ways to approach this problem.

Stratification

Perhaps the most intuitive approach to this problem is to build a model for each outcome. If there are 50 possible complications, we would create 50 logistic regression models to produce 50 probabilities (one for each complication type). While this type of modeling is a perfectly fine approach, there is a fair amount of overhead in the construction and (in the case of a deployed model) support of each model. Imagine if we wanted to stratify our models further to account for the unique risk associated with maternity and pediatric patients. Anaphylactic shock might be more relevant to pediatric patients, and eclampsia might be a complication more specific to maternity patients. Stratification in this way would certainly make clinical sense. However, for each outcome, we would have three substrata (maternity, pediatric, and other) and 150 models to develop and support. Yuck!

Stratification could also be employed for continuous outcomes. Perhaps we want to estimate patient cost within each revenue code (or cost bucket). Separate models could be developed for each cost type, but again, we must be cautious about the overhead with such an approach. While stratification is a valuable approach to account for the unique relationships between predictors (e.g., patient factors) and a response (e.g., outcome) within a particular stratum, the overhead involved in supporting such models should be considered. More sophisticated methods can be employed to estimate multiple continuous or binary outcomes. Rather than stratifying models based on each distinct outcome (e.g., complication types or revenue code-specific cost), we could consider a class of models specifically designed to model multiple responses.

Multinomial Regression

Multinomial regression is a general term used to describe regression models when the response variable has multiple categories (two or more) that are not ordered or hierarchical —that is, a *nominal* outcome. The base multinomial model requires that the outcomes being modeled are mutually exclusive. Only one of the outcomes is possible at a time. A variant of multinomial regression is multinomial logistic regression (MLR). This model would allow us to compute a probability for each distinct outcome. In our complications example, an MLR would enable us to develop a unified model that produces the probabilities for each outcome using the same set of predictor variables (or patient factors).

Here's a relevant code snippet in Python using `statsmodels`:

```
Multinomial: model = sm.MNLogit(df[['arrhythmias',
'pulmonary_edema', 'hypotension', 'infection']], X)
```

Likewise in R, using the nnet package:

```
model <- multinom(cbind(arrhythmias, pulmonary_edema,
hypotension, infection) ~ X, data = df)
```

In MLR, we model the probability that an observation falls into one of multiple categories or classes. The coefficients in the MLR represent the association between the predictor variables and the log odds of the different categories relative to a reference category.

These coefficients indicate how a one-unit change in that predictor variable is associated with the log odds of being in a particular category compared to the reference category.

The coefficients can be exponentiated to obtain an odds ratio to make the interpretation more intuitive. This ratio represents the multiplicative change in the odds of belonging to a specific category for a one-unit change in the predictor variable compared to the reference category. As with logistic regression (with a binary outcome), an odds ratio greater than 1 indicates an increase in the odds, while an odds ratio less than 1 indicates a decrease.

Multivariate Regression

In the case of the cost example, we could consider multivariate regression. This should not be confused with multiple (or multi-variable) regression referenced earlier in this chapter. Multivariate regression refers to a unified model with multiple continuous outcomes. In the cost example, we could generate an estimated cost for a patient for each revenue code ("room and board", "labs", "imaging", etc.) based on a single set of patient characteristics—comorbidities, complications, and procedures, perhaps.

A multivariate regression model typically has a set of coefficients for each outcome (response variable). Each outcome variable has its own set of coefficients associated with the predictor variables, which describe how each predictor variable affects each outcome variable.

For example, suppose we have three outcome variables (e.g., room and board, labs, and imaging) and four predictor variables (e.g., age, sex, ms-drg, and admission source). In that case, you will have a set of coefficients for each predictor variable for each outcome variable. This means that you'll have three sets of coefficients for room and board, three sets of coefficients for labs, and so on.

Since `statsmodels` does not support multiple response variables at the time of this book, we can use `sklearn` instead. Note that we have three response variables and three predictors in this excerpt of code, and therefore, we have three intercepts and three sets of coefficients.

```
from sklearn import linear_model
import pandas as pd
clf = linear_model.LinearRegression()
clf.fit(df[['room_and_board', 'labs',
'imaging']],df[['age','sex','ms_drg']])
print("Coefficients (Room and Board): "+ str(clf.
coef_[[0]]))
print("Intercept (Room and Board): " + str(clf.
intercept_[[0]]))
print("Coefficients (Labs): "+ str(clf.coef_[[1]]))
print("Intercept (Labs): " + str(clf.intercept_[[1]]))
print("Coefficients (Imaging): "+ str(clf.coef_[[2]]))
print("Intercept ("Imaging): " + str(clf.
intercept_[[2]]))
```

In R, we can simply use the lm() function. In the provided code, we fit a linear model where three response variables (room_and_board, labs, imaging) are modeled as a function of three predictors (age, sex, ms_drg). The cbind() function is used to combine the response variables into a matrix format, which can be used in the lm() function.

To extract the coefficients and their confidence intervals, we use the tidy() function from the broom package. This allows us to create a data frame of the model's coefficients. Have I mentioned that I love the broom package?

```
library(broom)
lm_model <- lm(cbind(room_and_board, labs, imaging) ~ age
+ sex + ms_drg, data = df)
coefficients_df <- tidy(lm_model, conf.int = TRUE)
print(coefficients_df)
```

Multi-Level Data

Quite often, the research question involves data at multiple levels. In my own research, this typically involves commingling hospital- and patient-level data. We must remember that not all predictor variables are equal in these cases and that the natural hierarchy of the data should be captured within the modeling effort, especially when we expect differences in variation within those levels.

Luckily, there is a flavor of regression specifically designed for these scenarios.

Mixed-effects models, often called hierarchical linear models or multilevel models, are a type of regression used to analyze data with a hierarchical or nested structure (or when there is natural clustering within-group levels).

Perhaps we are conducting a study related to patient cost, and we have a set of patient comorbidities and hospital characteristics (like teaching status, the urban or rural status of a hospital, or status as a level 1 trauma center) as predictor variables.

If we approached this problem using a mixed-effect model, we might classify the patient-level comorbidities as *fixed effects* while the hospital-level variables would be labeled as *random effects*. Sheesh, more terminology, Mike? Unfortunately, yes. Let's define some terms (it shouldn't be too painful). Fixed effects refer to variables that we want to estimate precisely. They are the specific variables that we want to estimate in our model (like the association between multiple sclerosis as a chronic condition and cost). In a fixed-effects model, we assume the effects are constant and apply to the entire population. Fixed effects are often the main factors we're interested in, and we estimate them with great accuracy.

On the other hand, *random effects* are a bit more nuanced. They represent sources of variability that you don't want to estimate precisely but rather account for in your model. Fixed effects are "fixed" and consistent throughout your data, while random effects are "random" sources of variation we're trying to model. Mixed-effects models allow one to incorporate both types of effects, providing a more accurate and flexible way to analyze complex data. However, these random effects must be categorical (not continuous). Including random effects can significantly improve the fit of your model, especially when you have nested or clustered data. Accounting for the inherent variability within levels makes the model more accurate and robust.

Tactically, the outcome of a mixed effect model produces coefficients for the fixed effects (as we have seen in the other models discussed in this chapter). However, with the random effects, the model produces separate intercepts for each random effect. In our cost example, we would have an intercept value for teaching status, urban/rural status, level 1 trauma status, etc.

Let's look at some notation:

$$Y = \alpha + \sum \beta_i X_i + \gamma + \varepsilon$$

where

Y is the response variable

α is the global intercept

β_i is set of fixed-effect coefficients corresponding to the predictor variables

X_i is a set of predictor variables. We use the summation symbol Σ (sigma) as a shorthand to summarize the predictor variables X_i weighted by their corresponding coefficients β_i. This keeps us from enumerating each predictor variable through the verbose subscripts.

γ represents a set of random effects. These can be thought of as intercepts specific to a higher-level grouping or cluster (e.g., hospital or physician-level characteristics).

The main difference between this notation and an OLS or Gaussian GLM is the inclusion of a set of random effects γ.

Now that we have provided some background on mixed effect models and presented the statistical notation, let's examine an example implementation in Python.

Again, we use the cost model discussed above for demonstration purposes.

Python

```
import numpy as np
import pandas as pd
import statsmodels.api as sm
import statsmodels.formula.api as smf
```

```
data = pd.DataFrame({
    'cost': [120, 130, 110, 140, 150, 130, 125, 135, 145,
155],
    'age': [45, 38, 52, 61, 33, 44, 56, 39, 50, 60],
    'sex': [1, 0, 1, 0, 1, 0, 1, 0, 1, 0],
    'arthritis': [1, 0, 0, 1, 0, 1, 0, 1, 1, 0],
    'ms': [0, 0, 1, 0, 1, 0, 0, 1, 0, 1],
    'kidney_disease': [1, 0, 0, 1, 0, 1, 0, 1, 0, 0],
    'diabetes': [0, 1, 0, 1, 0, 1, 0, 1, 0, 0],
    'teaching_status': [1, 0, 0, 1, 0, 1, 0, 1, 0, 0]
})

model = smf.mixedlm("cost ~ age + sex + arthritis
+ ms + kidney_disease + diabetes", data,
groups=data['teaching_status'])
result = model.fit()

print(result.summary())

fixed_effects = result.fe_params
random_effects = result.random_effects

print("\nFixed Effects:")
print(fixed_effects)

print("\nRandom Effects:")
print(random_effects)
```

Here, we are using the `mixedlm` method from `statsmodels`. Notice the designation of teaching status as a random effect using the group argument.

R
In R, lme4 is a well-supported package for mixed models:

```
library(lme4)

data <- data.frame(
    cost = c(120, 130, 110, 140, 150, 130, 125, 135, 145,
155),
    age = c(45, 38, 52, 61, 33, 44, 56, 39, 50, 60),
    sex = c(1, 0, 1, 0, 1, 0, 1, 0, 1, 0),
    arthritis = c(1, 0, 0, 1, 0, 1, 0, 1, 1, 0),
    ms = c(0, 0, 1, 0, 1, 0, 0, 1, 0, 1),
    kidney_disease = c(1, 0, 0, 1, 0, 1, 0, 1, 0, 0),
    diabetes = c(0, 1, 0, 1, 0, 1, 0, 1, 0, 0),
    teaching_status = c(1, 0, 0, 1, 0, 1, 0, 1, 0, 0)
)

model <- lmer(cost ~ age + sex + arthritis + ms + kidney_
disease + diabetes + (1 | teaching_status), data = data)
```

```
summary(model)

fixed_effects <- fixef(model)
print("\nFixed Effects:")
print(fixed_effects)

random_effects <- ranef(model)
print("\nRandom Effects:")
print(random_effects)
```

Using lme4, we indicate a random effect using the syntax (1 | teaching_status).

In both implementations, we extract the fixed and random effects from the result object; however, it is important to understand that random effects are used to account for variability at the group level and do not provide direct statistical measures such as confidence intervals, standard errors, or *p*-values, which are available for fixed effects (e.g., age, sex).

Zero-Inflated Response

In 2021, we collaborated with a local university on a problem related to ICD-10 coding intensity. If you read Chapter 2, you might remember this topic. There's no judgment if you skipped it. It was admittedly a fairly dry chapter.

In short, coding intensity refers to the thoroughness of coding ICD-10 codes using information from electronic health records. In one of those studies, we evaluated coding intensity by counting ICD-10 procedures as our response variable, conditioning on a patient, and hospital characteristics as predictor variables. Not all patients have a procedure conducted while in the hospital, so if we plot the distribution of patient procedure counts, we see a large proportion of zeros alongside another distribution (Poisson in this case). The distributional assumptions of regression were violated—even with the flexibility of a GLM. Figure 6.5 is an example of what a zero-inflated distribution might look like.

How do we model an outcome with two distinct groups within the response variable? Mike, at this point, shouldn't we consider gradient-boosted trees? Hold your horses, cowboy. It's time to talk about zero-inflated models.

Zero-inflated models are designed to specifically address this type of data using two components: a binary process and a counting process. The binary process is the part of the model that deals with whether a data point is zero. It

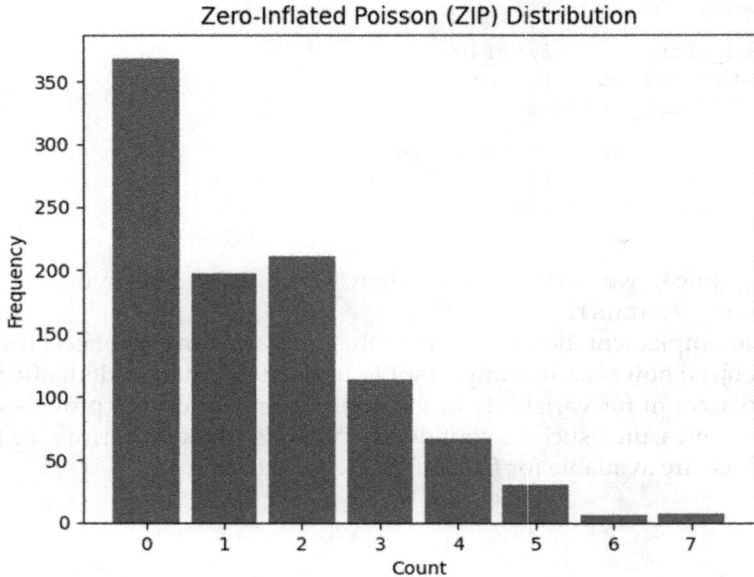

FIGURE 6.5
Example of a zero-inflated Poisson distribution

represents whether the event will happen or not. In our procedure example, it captures the probability of a procedure occurring. Once we've determined if the event will likely happen, the count process models the expected count of that response (e.g., the number of procedures). This part typically follows a distribution like Poisson or negative binomial, given that zero inflation typically occurs with count data.

Let's look at some notation.

$$Y \sim ZIP(\lambda, p)$$

where

Y represents the observed count data, typically following a Poisson distribution.

ZIP represents the zero-inflated Poisson (ZIP) model.

λ (lambda) is the parameter for the Poisson distribution. It represents the mean count when the count is not zero-inflated.

p indicates the probability that the observed count is zero due to an additional process other than the Poisson distribution.

We're cheating a bit here with the notation by abstracting away some of the statistical minutiae. The important part to communicate here is that two components are in play in a zero-inflated model—the probability of a zero and the parameter for the non-inflated distribution.

To demonstrate a ZIP model in Python using the response variable "number of procedures" and the predictor variables "age", "sex", and "MS-DRG", we can again use the statsmodels library. Here's an example:

```
import pandas as pd
import statsmodels.api as sm
import statsmodels.discrete.count_model as zip

data = {
    'Age': [45, 60, 50, 65, 55, 70, 65, 40, 70, 60, 45,
60, 50, 65, 55, 70, 65, 40, 70, 60],
    'Female':    [1, 0, 1, 0, 1, 1, 0, 1, 0, 1, 1, 0, 1,
0, 1, 1, 0, 1, 1, 1],
    'Diabetic':    [0, 1, 0, 1, 0, 1, 1, 0, 0, 0, 0, 1, 0,
1, 0, 1, 1, 0, 0, 1],
    'Procedures': [0, 5, 0, 2, 0, 0, 1, 0, 0, 4, 0, 6, 0,
3, 0, 0, 2, 0, 0, 0]
}
df = pd.DataFrame(data)
Y = df['Procedures']
X = df[["Age", "Female", "Diabetic"]]

model = zip.ZeroInflatedPoisson(Y, X, inflation='logit',
exog_infl=X)
results = model.fit()

print(results.summary())
```

In this example, we call ZeroInflatedPoisson from statsmodels. The inflation='logit' argument states that we want to use logistic regression to estimate the probability of a procedure before the Poisson model. The exog_infl=X argument states that we want to use the same predictors in the logistic model as in the subsequent Poisson model.

The results.summary() call provides information on the model's coefficients, standard errors, and other statistical details. Notice the two sets of coefficients for the two model stages (logistic and Poisson).

Similarly, we can use the pscl package in R to implement a ZIP model:

```
library(pscl)
data <- data.frame(
  Age = c(45, 60, 50, 65, 55, 70, 65, 40, 70, 60, 45, 60,
50, 65, 55, 70, 65, 40, 70, 60),
```

```
  Female = c(1, 0, 1, 0, 1, 1, 0, 1, 0, 1, 1, 0, 1, 0, 1,
1, 0, 1, 1, 1),
  Diabetic = c(0, 1, 0, 1, 0, 1, 1, 0, 0, 0, 0, 1, 0, 1,
0, 1, 1, 0, 0, 1),
  Procedures = c(0, 5, 0, 2, 0, 0, 1, 0, 0, 4, 0, 6, 0,
3, 0, 0, 2, 0, 0, 0)
)
zip_model <- zeroinfl(Procedures ~ Age + Female +
Diabetic, data = data, dist = "poisson")

summary(zip_model)
```

Interpreting the coefficients of a ZIP model is similar to interpreting coefficients in other regression models. Still, there are some unique considerations due to the two parts of the ZIP model: one part models the probability of observing a zero (the excess zeros, often modeled with logistic regression), and the other part models the count distribution (usually a Poisson distribution).

For each predictor variable in the logistic regression part, the coefficients represent the change in log odds of observing a zero count for a one-unit change in that predictor variable. A positive coefficient indicates an increase in the odds of observing a zero, while a negative coefficient indicates a decrease.

In the Poisson regression component, the coefficients for each predictor variable represent the change in the log of the expected count for a one-unit change in that predictor variable.

An exponentiated coefficient represents the multiplicative change in the expected count for a one-unit change in the predictor variable.

Other Data Scenarios

In my experience, the modeling strategies above address some of the most common data scenarios, especially when modeling an outcome against a set of patient characteristics. However, it is also important to mention a few less common scenarios (although they may be more common for your specific work). This section aims to inform the reader (you) that these models exist so that they can be pursued further in their own research if appropriate.

Response is Ordinal

A few years ago, I was part of a research team collaborating with a local university to provide some interpretability on how the CMS Overall Star

Hospital Ratings are associated with each measure used in the program. At the time, the CMS program used some opaque techniques (latent variable models and hierarchical clustering) to determine a hospital's star rating—an ordinal value ranging from 1 to 5. We aimed to provide more transparency by regressing the star rating (the response) directly on the hospital-level measure results (the predictors). The problem here is that ordinal variables are not always linear—that is, we cannot assume that the leap in performance from 1 star to another is the same despite the stars being ordered values.

Ordinal regression is a statistical analysis used when your response variable is ordered. In ordinal regression, the goal is to predict the likelihood of an observation falling into a particular category or a category below or above it based on one or more predictor variables. The key idea is to model the cumulative probabilities of the categories.

Python

Here's a code snippet of the model using OrderedLogit from statsmodels.

```
model = smf.OrderedLogit(endog=data[star_rating'],
exog=sm.add_constant(data['measure_value'])).fit()
print(model.summary)
```

R

And in R, we can use `polr` function in the MASS library:

```
library(MASS)
model <- polr(star_rating ~ measure_value, data = data)
Display the summary of the model
summary(model)
```

Interpreting the coefficients of an ordinal regression model requires some specific considerations for the ordinal nature of the response variable. The intercept represents the log odds of the cumulative probability of being in or below a particular category (usually the first) when all predictor variables are zero. This is the baseline category. For each predictor variable, a set of coefficients is produced for each category (excluding the last category). These coefficients indicate how a one-unit change in that predictor variable is associated with the log odds of being in a particular category compared to the previous category.

In ordinal regression, cut points or thresholds separate the different categories. These cut points determine the range of values for which the predicted probabilities correspond to a specific category. To make the interpretation more intuitive, the coefficients can again be exponentiated to yield odds ratios. An odds ratio represents the multiplicative change in the odds of moving to a higher category for a one-unit change in the predictor variable.

Outcome Is Dependent on Exposure or Observation Time

There are occasions when the outcome we're modeling depends on some baseline exposure or observation time. Representative examples can be seen with many healthcare-acquired infections (HAIs). HAIs have varying culture periods; therefore, the longer the exposure to certain conditions, the more likely an HAI is to occur.

Central line-associated bloodstream infections (CLABSIs), for example, are among the more common HAI examples. The risk of a bloodstream infection increases the longer the patient has a central line. As such, we should consider central line days as the "device days" specific to CLABSI. The number of days is the exposure or observation time we expect to increase the risk of a CLABSI.

In this hypothetical example, we might be evaluating facility-level HAI counts and want to understand if teaching hospitals are associated with higher incidences of HAIs. We could think of the outcome as the number of HAI incidences over the total device days $\frac{hai\,count}{exposure}$ (an incidence rate) while conditioning on an indicator for hospital teaching status. Modeling ratios directly is problematic because a zero in the numerator will result in a loss of information contained in our exposure. That is, we would be unable to distinguish 0 HAIs out of 100 days from 0 HAIs out of 1 day.

A rate regression can be used with a Poisson distribution in these scenarios, since count data is more common in these instances.

Python

To implement a Poisson rate regression in Python, in this case, we can specify the exposure time (e.g., central line days) as an offset variable in our standard GLM modeling. An excerpt of this implementation in Python can be seen as follows (using `statsmodels`):

```
offset = np.log(df[exposure])
model = sm.GLM(y, X, offset=offset, family=sm.families.
Poisson())
print(model)
```

R

In R, we can use base `glm` function:

```
model <- glm(y ~ age + sex + ms_drg, family = poisson(),
data = df, offset = log(exposure))
summary(model)
```

Expressed in notation, the applied model above takes the following form:

$$\log\left(\text{hai\_count}\right) = \alpha + \beta_1 \text{teaching}_1 + \log\left(\text{exposure}\right) + \varepsilon$$

Wait, Mike. That's not a rate you're modeling! Although it might not seem like it, we are using some tricky math with logarithms to model the outcome as a rate (i.e., $\frac{\text{hai count}}{\text{exposure}}$). Let's break it down a bit. With some simple algebra, we can move the exposure variable to the left-hand side of the equation as follows:

$$\log\left(\text{hai\_count}\right) - \log\left(\text{exposure}\right) = \alpha + \beta_1 \text{teaching}_1 + \varepsilon$$

If you recall from your beginner statistics class, subtraction in log form is equivalent to division, so we can express the same equation as follows:

$$\log\left(\frac{\text{hai\_count}}{\text{exposure}}\right) = \alpha + \beta_1 \text{teaching}_1 + \varepsilon$$

Voila! The offset is what allows us to calculate the incidence rate, hence the name "Poisson rate regression".

Handling Complex Interaction between Predictors

Interactions between predictors occur when one predictor has a conditional relationship on one or more other predictors. This can be problematic in regression, as our assumption of predictor independence is violated, leading to potentially misleading model coefficients.

If the set of predictor variables is manageable, we can create interaction terms for those predictors. For example, the risk of adverse events as a patient ages will differ by sex. Therefore, we might want to consider an interaction term between sex and age to inform the model of the relationship between age and sex.

When working with large sets of predictors with complex interactions, we end up in a bit of a pickle. Perhaps we're evaluating a broad set of comorbidities as predictor variables for a specific health outcome. It is very likely that some of those comorbidities, when present together, increase the risk of the outcome in a more complex manner (e.g., a complex causal system comprised of multiple related variables).

In this scenario, there are few great options with regression models (in my opinion), and it is worth exploring models that are structurally better suited for these scenarios. Tree-based , and methods like Structural Equation Modeling (SEM), models are helpful in these cases as they are conditional by nature; however, those methods are outside the scope of this book. Like regression, it is important to start with simple models (a simple decision tree) with the greatest level of interpretability and work toward more sophisticated approaches as needed. We might then employ a random forest model and ultimately delve into the world of gradient-boosted trees, if necessitated by the data. There are methods that provide some interpretability with these models when the data circumstances require it. For example, one may evaluate the SHapley Additive exPlanation (SHAP) values of an XGBoost model as an analog to odds ratios produced from a regression model. SHAP values are a powerful and interpretable tool for understanding the importance and contribution of individual features in machine learning models. They provide a way to explain the output of a model by attributing the prediction for a specific instance to each of its features.

Conclusion

There are many other modeling techniques that I've excluded in this chapter. For example, we have not touched on best subsets, piecewise regression, robust regression, weighted least squares, nonlinear regression, and a whole host of techniques that are not regression-based. Consider this section as the starter pack for regression analysis. This guide is designed for the beginner, and so as the reader becomes comfortable with these techniques, there are many great resources that provide more depth and breadth. I've listed some of my favorite resources at the end of this chapter for those interested in continuing further.

On the other hand, you may not ever want to hear the word regression again, and that's okay, too! Either way, the techniques discussed in this chapter will allow beginners to address the majority of everyday data problems. In my own work, it is uncommon for me to employ methods beyond those listed here—although it does happen from time to time.

If you're ready to throw in the towel, hang in there a bit longer. You've made it through the most challenging chapter. It is downhill from here!

Additional Resources

James, G., Witten, D., Hastie, T., & Tibshirani, R. (2021). *Introduction to Statistical Learning*. Springer. Available online: https://www.statlearning.com
Hastie, T., Tibshirani, R., & Friedman, J. (2009). *The Elements of Statistical Learning: Data Mining, Inference, and Prediction* (2nd ed.). Springer. Available online: https://hastie.su.domains/ElemStatLearn/

7

Measures of Disease Frequency and Association

This chapter covers two methods typically used to quantify disease frequency and association. While these topics are common across many healthcare disciplines, they are especially common in the field of epidemiology. There are many ways we might express the frequency of a disease and its association with specific exposures, and each method has advantages and disadvantages. Healthcare literature is often riddled with flowery, domain-specific language that can turn off many readers (despite the simplicity of many of the techniques being employed). Therefore, a secondary objective of this chapter is to explain these techniques from a layperson's perspective. A quick guide for some of the more common calculations is also included for easy reference (Table 7.1).

TABLE 7.1

Common Measures of Disease Frequency and Association

Term	Description	Calculation	Recommended Usage
Incidence Proportion	Proportion of new cases within	Incidence Proportion $= \dfrac{\text{Number of new cases}}{\text{Population at risk}}$	Captures the proportion of individuals who develop a condition within a specific population during a particular time frame.
Incidence Rate	Rate of occurrence of new cases	Incidence Rate $= \dfrac{\text{Number of new cases}}{\text{Person time at risk}}$	Useful in comparing disease occurrences among populations with different follow-up times or exposure durations.
Prevalence	Proportion of existing cases in a population	Prevalence $= \dfrac{\text{Number of existing cases}}{\text{Population at risk}}$	Indicates the total number of individuals affected by a disease or condition within a population at a specific point or over a period.

(Continued)

DOI: 10.1201/9781003609759-7

TABLE 7.1 (CONTINUED)

Term	Description	Calculation	Recommended Usage
Risk Ratio	Ratio of the probability of an event	Risk in exposed group $$= \frac{exposed\ cases}{all\ exposed}$$ Risk in unexposed group $$= \frac{unexposed\ cases}{all\ unexposed}$$ Risk Ratio $$= \frac{Risk\ in\ exposed\ group}{Risk\ in\ unexposed\ group}$$	Compares the probability of a disease in an exposed group to that in an unexposed group, indicating the strength of association between exposure and disease.
Risk Difference	Absolute difference in risks between groups	Risk Difference = Risk in exposed group – Risk in unexposed group	Measures the absolute difference in the probability of an disease between exposed and unexposed groups.
Odds Ratio	Odds of an event occurring in the exposed group relative to the unexposed group	Odds of event in exposed group $$= \frac{Exposed\ Cases}{Exposed\ Noncases}$$ Odds of event in unexposed group $$= \frac{Unexposed\ Cases}{Unexposed\ Noncases}$$ Odds Ratio $$= \frac{Odds\ of\ event\ in\ exposed\ group}{Odds\ of\ event\ in\ unexposed\ group}$$	Quantifies the odds of an event happening in an exposed group relative to the odds in an unexposed group, commonly used in case-control studies or logistic regression.

While the examples provided in this chapter demonstrate how the association between exposure and disease can be measured, I will stress that these methods have a broad utility beyond disease/exposure associations.

It will be helpful to define some terminology before we proceed with this chapter.

I've mentioned the term "exposure" several times already. Exposure in epidemiology refers to contact or interaction with some factor that could affect a person's health or lead to a particular disease or condition. "Exposure" might include elements such as infectious agents, chemicals, environmental factors, behaviors, or even genetic predispositions that might increase the risk of developing a particular disease or condition.

The terms *cases* and *controls* will also be used throughout this chapter. In epidemiology, *cases* refer to individuals with a particular disease or condition of interest. These individuals are the focus of the study as they already possess the health issue being studied. On the other hand, *controls* are individuals who do not have the disease or condition being investigated but are similar in various aspects to the cases. They serve as a comparison group, allowing researchers to analyze and compare factors such as exposures, behaviors, or other characteristics between the cases and controls.

Another important phrase is the *population at risk*, which refers to individuals susceptible to a particular disease, health condition, or event within a defined timeframe. It includes individuals who have not yet developed the condition but are at risk of doing so based on various factors such as age, gender, genetic predisposition, environmental, or lifestyle choices.

I'll also use the term *rate* and *proportion* regularly throughout this chapter. As a refresher, a proportion is a measure that represents a part of a whole, typically expressed as a fraction or percentage. It signifies the size or frequency of a subgroup within a larger group—for instance, the proportion of people in Union County, NC, with an active COVID-19 infection.

A rate assesses the frequency or occurrence of an event within a specific timeframe, often considering the population size or a standard unit of measurement. It's used to quantify changes or occurrences over time, such as the rate of catheter-associated bloodstream infections (CLABSIs) per catheter day. Rates provide information about events relative to the population size or a specified unit.

Measures of Disease Frequency

We'll begin this section by way of example. Let's say we're interested in understanding if bariatric surgery (weight loss surgery involving the stomach or intestines) is associated with osteoporosis (a disease resulting in decreased bone density). We might speculate that bariatric surgery may result in a nutritional deficiency and, therefore, decrease bone density. Table 7.2 has a mock study population of 3,500 individuals. We can refer to the 3,500 individuals as the *population at risk*—the number of people at risk for osteoporosis. Of this sample, five people had bariatric surgery and were diagnosed with osteoporosis, 40 had bariatric surgery and were not diagnosed with osteoporosis, 35 did not have

TABLE 7.2

An Example of a 2 × 2 Contingency Table

Exposure	New Cases (Osteoporosis)	Controls (No Osteoporosis)	Total
Had bariatric surgery	5	40	45
Did not have bariatric surgery	35	3,420	3,455
Total	40	3,460	3,500

bariatric surgery and were diagnosed with osteoporosis, and 3,420 did not have bariatric surgery and did not develop osteoporosis. All cases of osteoporosis were diagnosed within the study period (2023).

Incidence versus Prevalence

The term *incidence* (also referred to as *risk)* quantifies the new cases of a disease. In our dataset in Table 7.2, there are 40 incidence of osteoporosis. In this example, the *incidence proportion* of osteoporosis cases is calculated as the number of new cases over the population at risk:

$$\text{incidence proportion} = \frac{\text{new cases of osteoporosis}}{\text{population at risk}} = \frac{40}{3,500} = 0.0114$$

An alternative way to express incidence is through a rate, whereby the denominator is represented by person-years (the total number of years of life) rather than the number of people.

$$\text{incidence rate} = \frac{\text{new cases of osteoporosis}}{\text{person years at risk}}$$

Incidence values can be quite small (especially with rare diseases), so we often multiply them by a constant for better interpretation. In the incidence proportion example, 0.0114 x 1,000 would tell us that osteoporosis occurs in roughly 11.4 cases per 1,000 people (assuming a representative population sample).

Calculating incidences Python and R is one step beyond writing "Hello World". Here, we show the incidence proportion of osteoporosis cases for all individuals in our study:

Python

```
new_cases = 40
persons_at_risk = 3500
incidence = new_cases/persons_at_risk
print("Incidence Proportion:", incidence)
```

R

```
new_cases <- 40
persons_at_risk <- 3500
incidence <- new_cases / persons_at_risk
print(paste("Incidence Proportion:", incidence))
```

Prevalence, another measure of disease frequency, refers to the proportion of disease cases in a population at a given point in time. It differs from incidence in that it does not require the cases to be newly identified within the study period. In the osteoporosis example, prevalence would include all active cases, including those identified during the study period and those existing before the study period.

The code is easy-peasy. Perhaps nine people had osteoporosis before the beginning of our study period. In this case, there would be nine existing cases and 40 new cases, totaling 49 cases of osteoporosis:

Python

```
existing_cases = 49
total_population = 3500
prevalence = (existing_cases / total_population) * 100
print("Prevalence:", prevalence, "%")
```

R

```
existing_cases <- 49
total_population <- 3500
prevalence <- (existing_cases / total_population) * 100
print(paste("Prevalence:", prevalence, "%"))
```

Prevalence is measured as a proportion (e.g., the proportion of people with diabetes among the total population), which provides a snapshot of how widespread a condition is at a particular moment. It's a static measure that estimates the disease or condition's burden within the population.

A common analogy to distinguish incidence and prevalence involves a bathtub with a dripping faucet (Figure 7.1).

In the bathtub analogy, the capacity of the bathtub represents the population at risk, and the water in the tub represents the proportion of the population with the disease at a given time. An individual may recover from the disease (the evaporation of the water in this analogy) or expire (a leak from the bottom of the tub). New cases in the population at risk are identified through the drops from the dripping faucet.

While new cases of the disease (incidence) increase prevalence, death and recovery decrease prevalence. As a result, we can see that prevalence is constantly fluctuating. We might even say that prevalence is a *fluid* measure. I'll see myself out.

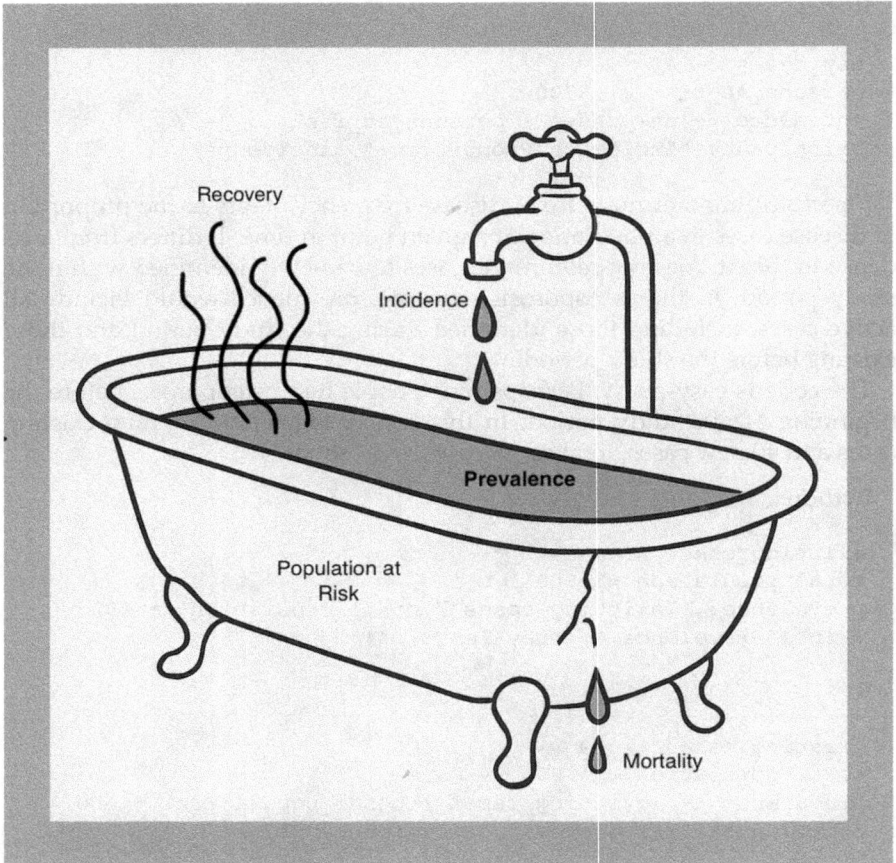

FIGURE 7.1
A bathtub analogy illustrating the relationship between incidence, prevalence, recovery, mortality, and population at risk.

Measures of Association

Measures of association allow us to quantify the relationship between an exposure (e.g., bariatric surgery) and a disease (osteoporosis). These are simple but incredibly powerful tools that I personally use quite often in everyday healthcare analyses. In this section, we'll cover three important techniques: (1) Odds Ratios, (2) Risk Ratios, and (3) Risk Difference. While these are similar methods, they each have distinct advantages and disadvantages.

Before we begin, let's review the fine print: These methods will not provide causal information. While the two factors might be associated, we cannot say that one is necessarily the cause of the other (there is a burgeoning field of statistics designed to identify causal relationships). These methods provide important directional information that may support the need to conduct further research using more robust methods (such as causal analysis).

As a further disclaimer, the motivating example used in this chapter assumes that there are no confounding variables (this is not often the case in real-world analysis). The chapter on regression methods discusses controlling for confounding variables. We also assume that our data is a representative sample of the population and, therefore, is not biased by the selection of participants. Finally, the examples are provided simply to demonstrate the techniques and not to share any real-world clinical findings.

Risk Ratios

We'll start with the concept of a risk—which is simply the proportion of the event in a group. We could refer to this as a crude probability of an event. The risk of osteoporosis for patients having bariatric surgery is as follows:

$$\text{risk exposed} = \frac{\text{cases exposed}}{\text{all exposed}} = \frac{5}{45} = 0.111$$

Similarly, the risk of osteoporosis for patients who did not undergo bariatric surgery is calculated as follows:

$$\text{risk unexposed} = \frac{\text{cases unexposed}}{\text{all unexposed}} = \frac{35}{3,455} = 0.010$$

Therefore, the risk ratio (also called relative risk) is the ratio of the probability of an event occurring in an exposed group to the probability in an unexposed group. It measures the strength of the association between exposure and disease.

Again, in the context of our osteoporosis example, the *risk ratio* is calculated by dividing the risk in the unexposed group from the risk in the exposed group:

$$\text{risk ratio} = \frac{\text{risk exposed}}{\text{risk unexposed}} = \frac{\text{cases exposed}}{\text{all exposed}} \div \frac{\text{cases unexposed}}{\text{all unexposed}}$$

$$11.1 = \frac{0.111}{0.010} = \frac{5}{45} \div \frac{35}{3,455}$$

The interpretation of a risk ratio is simple. A risk ratio greater than 1 indicates that exposure is associated with an increased disease risk. In contrast, a risk ratio of less than 1 means that the exposure is associated with a decreased disease risk (a protective effect). Risk ratios of 1 or near 1 indicate that the exposure is not associated with the risk of the disease.

A risk ratio of 11.1 means that individuals having bariatric surgery have over 11 times the risk of developing osteoporosis compared to individuals not having bariatric surgery (assuming that the individuals are alike in every other way).

We can write this code with our eyes closed.

Python

```
exposed_cases = 5
exposed_noncases = 40
unexposed_cases = 35
unexposed_noncases = 3455

RR = (exposed_cases / (exposed_cases + exposed_
noncases)) / (unexposed_cases / (unexposed_cases +
unexposed_noncases))
print("Relative Risk (RR):", RR)
```

R

```
exposed_cases <- 5
exposed_noncases <- 40
unexposed_cases <- 35
unexposed_noncases <- 3455

RR <- (exposed_cases / (exposed_cases + exposed_
noncases)) / (unexposed_cases / (unexposed_cases +
unexposed_noncases))
print(paste("Relative Risk (RR):", RR))
```

Note that we can also evaluate a ratio of rates (rather than proportions) to form a risk rate ratio. The interpretation of a risk rate ratio is the same as a risk ratio in that we are measuring the increased rate of an event in one group relative to another.

Odds Ratios

Just as we defined risk before discussing risk ratios, we must define odds before discussing odds ratios. Odds are defined as a ratio of the number of cases to non-cases and represent the likelihood of an event happening. In the osteoporosis example, the odds of osteoporosis would be calculated as follows:

$$\text{odds of osteoporosis} = \frac{\text{cases}}{\text{non cases}} = \frac{40}{3,460}$$

We could also calculate the odds of osteoporosis for individuals with bariatric surgery $\frac{5}{40} = 0.125$ or the odds of osteoporosis for individuals not having bariatric surgery $\frac{35}{3,420} = 0.010$.

Odds *ratios* are designed to evaluate the odds of exposure among cases compared to controls, helping to measure the strength of association. We don't need a detective to figure out that the odds ratio is simply a ratio of the odds of an event occurring in one group to the odds of it happening in another group.

$$\text{odds ratio} = \frac{\text{odds of osteoporosis for bariatric surgery patients}}{\text{odds of osteoporosis for non bariatric surgery patients}}$$

The interpretation of an odds ratio is similar to that of a risk ratio. Odds ratios greater than 1 indicate that exposure is associated with higher odds of acquiring the disease, while odds ratios less than 1 indicate that exposure is associated with lower odds of acquiring the disease. Odds ratios of 1 or near 1 indicate no association between exposure and disease.

In this mock example, the odds of having osteoporosis are 12.21 times higher for individuals having bariatric surgery compared to those not having bariatric surgery. In other words, individuals having bariatric surgery were 12.21 times more likely to develop osteoporosis compared to those without surgery (assuming all other characteristics are the same).

$$12.21 = \frac{5}{40} \div \frac{35}{3,420}$$

The Python implementation is a piece of cake:

```
exposed_cases = 5
exposed_non_cases = 40

unexposed_cases = 35
unexposed_non_cases = 3420

OR = (exposed_cases * unexposed_non_cases) / (exposed_
non_cases * unexposed_cases)
print("Odds Ratio (OR):", OR)
```

As is with R:

```
exposed_cases <- 5
exposed_non_cases <- 40
```

```
unexposed_cases <- 35
unexposed_non_cases <- 3420

OR <- (exposed_cases * unexposed_non_cases) / (exposed_
non_cases * unexposed_cases)
print(paste("Odds Ratio (OR):", OR))
```

Note that it is common to see an alternative odds ratio calculation written as follows (which is mathematically equivalent to the previous formula):

$$\text{odds ratio} = \frac{\text{exposed cases} \times \text{unexposed non cases}}{\text{exposed non cases} \times \text{unexposed cases}}$$

$$12.21 = \frac{5 \times 3,420}{40 \times 35}$$

If you're still struggling with the difference between odds and risk ratios, Figure 7.2 has been provided to help visualize the difference between an odds ratio and risk ratio using a set of 19 individuals. I'll credit Josh Starmer from StatQuest (one of my favorite statistics educators), whose book inspired these visualizations. Triple bam!

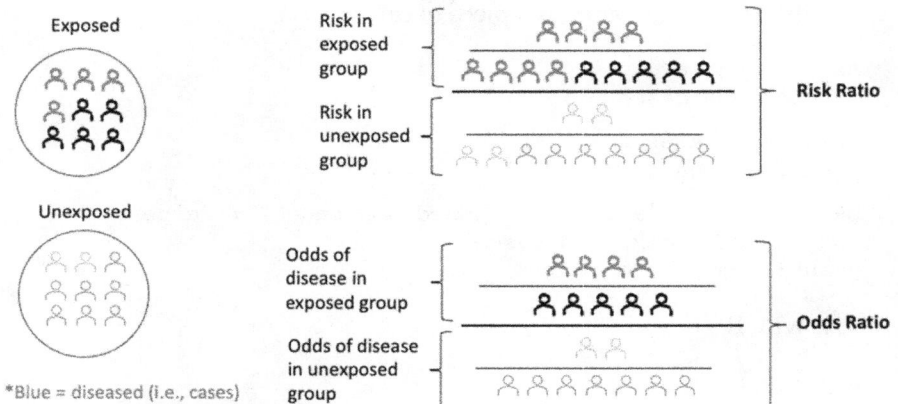

FIGURE 7.2
A comparison between risk ratio and odds ratio calculations.

Risk Difference

Risk difference is a measure of absolute effect. The difference in risk between exposed and unexposed groups represents the proportion of cases attributable to the exposure. The *risk difference* is therefore calculated by subtracting the risk in the unexposed group from the risk in the exposed group:

$$\text{risk difference} = \text{risk exposed} - \text{risk unexposed}$$

In the context of our osteoporosis example, the risk for the exposed population is the proportion of individuals having bariatric surgery who developed osteoporosis, and the risk for the unexposed population is the proportion of individuals who did not have bariatric surgery who developed osteoporosis.

$$11.5\% = 12.5\% - 1.0\% = \frac{5}{40} - \frac{35}{3,455}$$

The 11.5% risk difference between the bariatric surgery group and the non-bariatric surgery group demonstrates that the bariatric surgery group is associated with an increased risk of osteoporosis by 11.5 percentage points.

Relative risk represents the absolute change in the probability of an event occurring due to an exposure or an intervention. While risk ratios and risk difference are a necessary component in understanding the impact of exposures or interventions, they focus on different aspects of the relationship between exposure and disease. Risk difference measures the absolute change in risk, while risk ratios quantify the ratio of risks between groups.

Choosing between Relative Risk and Odds Ratios

Odds and risk ratios are quite similar, and each has advantages and disadvantages. The choice between them often depends on the characteristics of the study and the data itself. I personally prefer to use odds ratios when doing regression analysis with a binary response (e.g., a disease or outcome). Oftentimes, I like to show the unadjusted odds ratio for some person characteristic alongside an adjusted odds ratio, to show how the ratio changes when controlling for other confounding variables.

For example, we might construct a table of predictors in a logistic regression model estimating osteoporosis as the response with multiple confounders. Recall that we can exponentiate the coefficients in a logistic regression to obtain an odds ratio (controlling for other confounding variables in the model). We can show an unadjusted odds ratio alongside the adjusted odds ratio from the

TABLE 7.3

Example Analysis Output Comparing Unadjusted and Adjusted Odds Ratios

	Unadjusted			Adjusted		
	OR	OR 95% CI	*p*-value	OR	OR 95% CI	*p*-value
Bariatric Surgery	12.21	7.59–9.33	.0610	8.46	7.59–9.33	.00319

logistic regression (Table 7.3). The compatibility of the odds ratio with logistic regression is why I prefer using them for binary regression analyses.

However, one drawback to odds ratios is that they are a bit harder to interpret. When speaking with a clinical stakeholder, I feel the more intuitive metric is the risk ratio (this is ultimately a matter of personal preference). Providing that the analysis is not part of a larger regression analysis, I prefer to use risk ratios.

There is a much more nuanced debate about when to use odds ratios and risk ratios, and additional resources are provided at the end of this chapter for more information. Of course, it is always helpful to provide multiple statistics to provide a more complete picture of the data scenario. For example, we might include the raw count data, risk difference, and risk ratio in our analyses to show the magnitude of the difference (using the risk difference) and the strength of the association (through the risk ratio). Remember, there is no singular value that will tell the whole story.

Statistical Significance

Okay Mike, I've calculated an odds ratio of 1.56 in my analysis. Is there an association between my exposure and outcome? Good question.

Just as there was a sampling error when comparing means or proportions in the chapter on hypothesis testing, odds ratios and risk ratios have similar characteristics. That is, evaluating an odds or risk ratio on its own will ultimately require a subjective interpretation from the stakeholder. We don't want that, of course, so we can use hypothesis testing again!

To evaluate the statistical significance of such associations we can formulate our hypothesis as follows:

Null Hypothesis:

There exposure is not associated with the disease (i.e., OR = 1)

Alternate Hypothesis:

There exposure is associated with the disease (i.e., OR ≠ 1)

As you might notice, we are conducting a two-sided test—testing for differences in either direction—however, left and right-tailed tests can also be calculated depending on the research question.

There are a variety of methods to determine the statistical significance of association; however, we'll focus on the Wald test.

Let's talk about these methods in more detail.

Wald Method

In the chapter on regression methods, we discussed the calculation of odds ratios from a logistic regression by exponentiating the coefficient (i.e., the logg odds). Recall also that we conducted a significance test on these coefficients to determine if the slope was 0. This approach, called the *Wald method*, is often used to estimate confidence intervals and test the statistical significance of parameters, including odds and risk ratios. The method involves dividing the estimated coefficient (e.g., odds ratio or risk ratio) by its standard error to obtain a z-score. This z-score is then compared to the standard normal distribution to determine statistical significance. This test is best applied when the sample size is large enough to approximate a normal distribution accurately. Therefore, caution should be exercised when the sample size is small.

We can conveniently use the GLM framework to calculate an odds ratio and test its significance against some predetermined confidence level (e.g., 95%). The example below essentially regresses the disease on the exposure to obtain a regression coefficient. Using this method, we can extract the *p*-value for the exposure coefficient to determine if the association is significant at our desired significance level.

Python

```
import pandas as pd
import numpy as np
import statsmodels.api as sm

data = pd.DataFrame({
    'exposure': [0, 1, 0, 1, 1, 0, 0, 0],
    'disease': [0, 1, 0, 1, 0, 0, 1, 0]
})

data['intercept'] = 1

X = data[['intercept', 'exposure']]
y = data['disease']

model = sm.Logit(y, X)
result = model.fit()

odds_ratio = np.exp(result.params['exposure'])
wald_p_value = result.pvalues['exposure']

print(f"Odds Ratio: {odds_ratio}")
print(f"Wald Test P-value: {wald_p_value}")
```

R

```
data <- data.frame(
  exposure = c(0, 1, 0, 1, 1, 0, 0, 0),
  disease = c(0, 1, 0, 1, 0, 0, 1, 0)
)

model <- glm(disease ~ exposure, data = data, family =
binomial)

odds_ratio <- exp(coef(model)['exposure'])
wald_p_value <- summary(model)$coefficients['exposure',
'Pr(>|z|)']

cat(sprintf("Odds Ratio: %.4f\n", odds_ratio))
cat(sprintf("Wald Test P-value: %.4f\n", wald_p_value))
```

Confidence Intervals

Just as we can calculate confidence intervals for means and proportions, we can also calculate confidence intervals for odds ratios and risk ratios. The structure of the confidence interval is the same as those discussed in Chapter 4; however, how we define the standard error is unique to the measure of association. Since odds ratios and risk ratios cannot be below zero but can be any number greater than zero, the distributions for these measures are skewed right. Luckily, however, the distributions are log-normal, and so with a log transformation, we can assume that they follow a normal (or Gaussian) distribution. This type of transformation gives us the flexibility to use more direct and interpretable methods.

Confidence Intervals for Risk Ratios

We'll start with risk ratios. Recall that the critical z value and the standard error form the margin of error that is added and subtracted from the value of interest to form the confidence interval. Again, we are using the log of the risk ratio so the confidence intervals will also be on the log scale.

$$\left(CI_{lower}, CI_{upper}\right) = ln\left(\text{relative risk}\right) \pm z_{a/2} \times s.e.$$

The standard error formula is below. In short, this formula estimates the standard deviation of the natural logarithm of the risk ratio. It quantifies the uncertainty or variability in the risk ratio estimate due to the sample data.

$$s.e. = \sqrt{\frac{1 - \hat{p}_{exposed}}{n_{exposed}\hat{p}_{exposed}} + \frac{1 - \hat{p}_{unexposed}}{n_{unexposed}\hat{p}_{unexposed}}}$$

The standard error formula uses the proportion of cases for the exposed and unexposed groups, respectively.

$$\hat{p}_{\text{exposed}} = \frac{\text{exposed cases}}{\text{exposed cases} + \text{exposed noncases}}$$

$$\hat{p}_{\text{unexposed}} = \frac{\text{unexposed cases}}{\text{unexposed cases} + \text{unexposed noncases}}$$

In the context of the bariatric surgery and osteoporosis example, we can demonstrate the calculations:

$$s.e. = .1422 = \sqrt{\frac{1 - \frac{5}{45}}{45 \frac{5}{45}} + \frac{1 - \frac{35}{3,455}}{3,455 \frac{35}{3,455}}}$$

$$(2.1283, 2.686) = 2.407 \pm 1.96 \times .1422$$

Since we're working with logs, the natural log of 11.1 is 2.407, resulting in a margin of error of .2787 (or 1.96 × .1442). We use a critical z value of 1.96 for a 95% confidence interval.

The upper and lower confidence intervals must be exponentiated as follows to return them to their original scale:

$$(8.401, 14.673) = \left(e^{2.1283}, e^{2.686} \right)$$

With this information, we state that we are 95% confident that the true risk ratio is between 8.401 and 14.673.

In Python, we can compute the confidence interval as follows:

```python
import numpy as np

ln_risk_ratio = 0.779  # Natural logarithm of the
risk_ratio
z_critical = 1.96
confidence interval

p_hat_1 = 0.3
n_1 = 200
p_hat_2 = 0.2
n_2 = 200

se_ln_rr = np.sqrt((1 - p_hat_1) / (n_1 * p_hat_1) +
(1 - p_hat_2) / (n_2 * p_hat_2))

ci_low = ln_risk_ratio + z_critical * se_ln_rr * -1
ci_upp = ln_risk_ratio + z_critical * se_ln_rr

print(f"95% CI for ln(Relative Risk): ({ci_low:.3f},
{ci_upp:.3f})")
```

Similarly, in R:

```
ln_risk_ratio <- 0.779  # Natural logarithm of the risk
ratio
z_critical <- 1.96

p_hat_1 <- 0.3
n_1 <- 200
p_hat_2 <- 0.2
n_2 <- 200

se_ln_rr <- sqrt((1 - p_hat_1) / (n_1 * p_hat_1) + (1 -
p_hat_2) / (n_2 * p_hat_2))

ci_low <- ln_risk_ratio - z_critical * se_ln_rr
ci_upp <- ln_risk_ratio + z_critical * se_ln_rr

cat(sprintf("95%% CI for ln(Relative Risk): (%.3f,
%.3f)\n", ci_low, ci_upp))
```

Confidence Intervals for Odds Ratios

For odds ratios, the approach is similar. Again, we use the log of the odds ratios and add the margin of error on both sides of the log odds ratio.

$$\left(CI_{\text{lower}}, CI_{\text{upper}}\right) = ln\left(\text{odds ratio}\right) \pm z_{a/2} \times s.e.$$

We can approximate the standard error for the odds ratio using the raw values from each quadrant of our 2 × 2 contingency table, with *a–d* being read left to right and top to bottom.

$$s.e. = \sqrt{\frac{1}{a} + \frac{1}{b} + \frac{1}{c} + \frac{1}{d}}$$

A worked example using the bariatric surgery and osteoporosis example is as follows:

$$s.e. = 0.289 = \sqrt{\frac{1}{5} + \frac{1}{40} + \frac{1}{35} + \frac{1}{3,420}}$$

$$\left(1.945, 3.058\right) = 2.502 \pm 1.96 \times 0.289$$

With 2.502 as the natural log of the odds ratio of 12.21, we can calculate a margin of error of .2787 (or 1.96 × .1442) for a 95% confidence interval.

Again, the upper and lower confidence intervals must be exponentiated as follows to return them to their original scale:

$$\left(6.994, 21.285\right) = \left(e^{1.945}, e^{3.058}\right)$$

With this information, we state that we are 95% confident that the true odds ratio is between 6.994 and 21.285.

The Python implementation looks like this:

```
import numpy as np

a = 5
b = 40
c = 35
d = 3420

odds_ratio = (a * d) / (b * c)

z_critical = 1.96  # For a 95% confidence interval

se_ln_or = np.sqrt(1 / a + 1 / b + 1 / c + 1 / d)

ln_odds_ratio = np.log(odds_ratio)

ci_low = ln_odds_ratio + z_critical * se_ln_or * -1
ci_upp = ln_odds_ratio + z_critical * se_ln_or

print(f"95% CI for ln(Odds Ratio): ({ci_low:.3f},
{ci_upp:.3f})")
```

The R implementation looks like this:

```
a <- 5
b <- 40
c <- 35
d <- 3420

odds_ratio <- (a * d) / (b * c)

z_critical <- 1.96  # For a 95% confidence interval

se_ln_or <- sqrt(1 / a + 1 / b + 1 / c + 1 / d)

ln_odds_ratio <- log(odds_ratio)

ci_low <- ln_odds_ratio - z_critical * se_ln_or
ci_upp <- ln_odds_ratio + z_critical * se_ln_or

cat(sprintf("95%% CI for ln(Odds Ratio): (%.3f, %.3f)\n",
ci_low, ci_upp))
```

Effect Modification

We are making a bold assumption with our odds ratio and risk ratio calculation in that we are assuming that the association (e.g., bariatric surgery and osteoporosis) is consistent across person characteristics such as age, sex, and

TABLE 7.4

Contingency Table Stratified by Age to Test for Effect Modification

Exposure	Had bariatric surgery		Did not have bariatric surgery	
Stratum	New Cases (Osteoporosis)	Controls (No Osteoporosis)	New Cases (Osteoporosis)	Controls (No Osteoporosis)
Age 65+	3	16	14	1,368
Age 18–64	2	24	21	2,052

social circumstances. Of course, we can attempt to control for these factors through regression analyses (as discussed in the previous chapter); however, we might be interested in surfacing how the association changes for a specific factor (or level). The term for an association changing based on stratification or grouping by a specific variable, such as age, is called "effect modification" or "interaction". Effect modification occurs when the magnitude or direction of an association between an exposure and a disease (measured by the odds ratio, risk ratio, etc.) differs across different levels or strata.

It means that the relationship between the exposure and the disease is not consistent across all subgroups, and that the effect of the exposure may be modified by the stratifying variable (e.g., age, gender, or other factors).

Perhaps we want to know if the association between bariatric surgery and osteoporosis differs between individuals 18–65 and those 65 and older. To support these analyses, we've stratified the 2 × 2 table from the beginning of this chapter into two age groups (18–64 and 65+) in Table 7.4.

Breslow-Day Test

In the previous section, we introduced effect modification, where the strength of association between an exposure and outcome differs across levels of a third variable, such as age. To formally test whether these differences in association are statistically meaningful, we can use the Breslow-Day test for homogeneity of odds ratios.

The code below demonstrates how to test for effect modification using the statsmodels package in Python. We compare two age groups (18–65 and 65+) and assess whether the odds ratios for an exposure–outcome relationship (e.g., bariatric surgery and osteoporosis) are consistent across these strata.

```
import numpy as np
from statsmodels.stats.contingency_tables import
StratifiedTable

table_age_18_65 = np.array([[3, 16], [14, 1368]])
table_age_65_plus = np.array([[2, 24], [21, 2052]])
```

```
ctable = np.array([table_age_18_65, table_age_65_plus])

st = StratifiedTable(ctable)

test_result = st.test_equal_odds()

print("Breslow-Day Test for Homogeneity of Odds Ratios:")
print(f"Test Statistic: {test_result.statistic:.4f}")
print(f"P-value: {test_result.pvalue:.4f}")
```

Similarly in R, we can use the BreslowDayTest function in the DescTools library.

```
library(DescTools)

counts <- c(3,16,14,1368,  2,24,21,2052)

ctable <- array(counts, dim = c(2,2,2),
          dimnames = list(
            Exposure = c("Yes", "No"),
            Outcome = c("Case", "Control"),
            Stratum = c("18_65", "65_plus")
            ))

BreslowDayTest(ctable)
```

The Breslow-Day test for homogeneity of odds ratios evaluates whether the relationship between an exposure and an outcome differs across strata, such as different age groups. A p-value less than 0.05 indicates significant effect modification, meaning the odds ratios for the exposure-outcome association are different across the strata. This suggests that the exposure has a varying impact depending on the subgroup (e.g., age group). Conversely, a p-value greater than 0.05 implies no significant difference in odds ratios across strata. The test statistic quantifies the magnitude of difference between the odds ratios, with a higher value reflecting a greater disparity between the groups.

Conclusion

Congratulations! You've made it to the end of this chapter and now (hopefully) have a better grasp on how to quantify disease frequency and its association with an exposure variable. Additionally, my hope is that the reader is better equipped with the domain-specific terminology used to discuss disease frequency and association.

I will say that while the methods discussed in this chapter are often applied to some exposure and a resulting disease (or outcome), they are also incredibly useful in other aspects of healthcare analysis. For example, a few years ago, I was part of a team researching how we might make an informed decision on how to attribute physicians to patients, with the goal of identifying physicians who are most responsible for patient care during their inpatient stay (remember this discussion in chapter 2?). In this research, we used an odds ratio to identify the strength of association between the patient's MS-DRG (or disease group) and the physician's specialty to identify the physicians providing care most associated with the patient's principal diagnosis. We've also used measures of association to identify the complications that should be attributed to physicians based on their specialty. Furthermore, we've used odds ratios to identify resources that are relevant to certain physician's specialties (e.g., knee transplants are associated with orthopedic surgeons). As is the case with all methods discussed in this book, the reader is encouraged to consider the broader utility of these methods beyond the specific examples provided here.

Like many disciplines, we've only scratched the surface on this topic, and there is considerable depth in each of the topics discussed. Additional resources have been provided at the end of this chapter, along with a quick reference guide for many of the calculations discussed above.

As mentioned in the preface, I personally prefer simple methods when possible, and odds and risk ratios are fantastic tools for communicating with business and clinical stakeholders. Oftentimes, the results from these methods lead to more robust analyses, whereby additional confounding variables are considered to ensure the preliminary findings using odds ratios or risk ratios are corroborated by more robust methods.

In the next chapter, we will dig into the concept of risk standardization, a set of statistical tools that can pair nicely with the methods discussed in this chapter and others within this book

Additional Resources

Szklo, M., & Nieto, F. J. (2018). *Epidemiology: Beyond the Basics* (4th ed.). Jones & Bartlett Learning.

Lash, T. L., VanderWeele, T. J., Haneuse, S., & Rothman, K. J. (2021). *Modern Epidemiology* (4th ed.). LWW.

8

Standardization

The story you are about to hear is based on actual events; however, the names and data have been changed to protect the innocent. <queue the dramatic background music>

The adult death rate in Elder County, FL, is 0.0297, or approximately 29.7 deaths out of every 1,000 people. Now, this is a concerning number, especially given that the national death rate of all U.S. residents is .0166, or approximately 16.6 out of every 1,000 people. How can this be? Perhaps there was a rare, localized outbreak of some mysterious virus? Maybe it was a severe hurricane that struck the area? Perhaps there was a chemical leak that infected the water supply? Whatever it was, it was catastrophic, causing a death rate nearly double that of the national population. Something is wrong here, and we, as health researchers, must crack the case.

Sarah, the new Public Health intern, is tasked with unraveling this mystery. As she begins to dig into the data, she observes that there is no sudden spike in mortality occurring at some seminal event. In fact, the mortality rates are relatively stable each year. Nothing in the data appears to be out of the ordinary. Hours later, crunching code into the night hours in her cubical, she has an epiphany: The people of Elder County, FL, are old—really old. She shares a table with the percentage of residents by age group in Elder County compared to the national population (Table 8.1):

Given that the proportion of individuals 65+ is more than double that of the national population and the proportion of individuals 18–25 is less than half of the national population, it is no surprise that Elder County has a drastically higher mortality rate.

The *crude rate, which* considers the total number of events as a proportion of the population within some interval, is 29.7 deaths out of every 1,000 people. While the crude rate is helpful within the population being studied, it is a fairly lousy metric to use comparatively. Populations are not homogenous, so a direct comparison of crude rates can often be misleading (as demonstrated in this example).

In this chapter, we'll discuss *standardization*, a handy statistical tool that allows us to fairly compare groups fairly despite their differing compositions

DOI: 10.1201/9781003609759-8

TABLE 8.1

Age Distribution in Elder County, FL,
Compared to the National Population

Age Range Description	Age Range	Elder County	National
Young Adult	18–25	10%	24%
Adult	26–44	13%	25%
Middle Age	45–59	16%	23%
Old Age	60+	61%	28%

(within limits, of course). Specifically, we'll discuss two types of standardization: *direct* and *indirect*. We'll also discuss how the latter method can be used to evaluate the quality and efficiency of care while accounting for the varying distributions of patient and hospital characteristics within those populations. Cliffhanger: This is my favorite topic in the entire book.

Direct Standardization

Let's start with direct standardization. Direct standardization allows us to fairly compare two or more populations that differ in age distribution (or other characteristics of interest). To do this, we use knowledge of the broader, more representative, *standard population* (e.g., the United States) to adjust the event rates of interest within the narrower *target population* of interest (e.g., Elder County, FL). This adjustment aims to make fair comparisons across groups by creating a *standardized rate* or measure that eliminates (or minimizes) the effect of the differing population structures.

The general concept of *direct standardization* is that we reweight the age-specific rates in the target population based on the proportion of individuals in the standard population. In this example, the directly standardizing rates are achieved by weighting the age-specific crude death rate of Elder County by the proportion of patients in that age group within the larger U.S. population (the "standard population"). The result is a weighted average of the death rates (with the weights derived from the standard population).

Let's work through an example.

As shown in Table 8.2, the age imbalance between Elder County and the national population is clear. We can also see that when directly standardizing the mortality rate, the death rate for Elder County changes from 0.02968 (the crude rate) to .01513. Let's discuss the notation to produce a directly standardized rate in conceptual terms and then work through the example to see how we obtained the directly standardized rate of .01513.

TABLE 8.2

Example Calculation of Direct Standardization of Mortality Rates in Elder County, FL, Based on the Age Distribution of the National Population

Age Range Description	Standard Population		Target Population			
	Population (U.S.)	Proportion of Population (U.S.)	Population (Elder)	Deaths (Elder)	Death Rate (Elder)	Proportion (U.S.) × Death Rate (Elder)
Young Adult	43,327,382	0.23941	6,524	5	0.0008	0.00106
Adult	45,660,395	0.25230	8,698	22	0.0025	0.00063
Middle Age	40,994,370	0.22652	10,148	48	0.0047	0.00106
Old age	50,992,996	0.28177	39,142	1,840	0.047	0.01324
Total	180,975,143	1	64,512	1,915	0.02968	**0.01513**

(arrow pointing to 0.01513) Directly Standardized Death Rate (Elder)

The formula to produce the directly standardized rate takes the following form:

$$\text{Directly Standardized Rate} = \sum_{i=1}^{n}\left[\frac{\text{event count}_i^T}{\text{population size}_i^T} \times \frac{\text{population size}_i^S}{\sum \text{population size}_i^S} \right]$$

In short, this formula shows that for each age stratum i, we are weighting age-specific death rates within Elder County by the proportion of individuals within the same age stratum in the U.S. population. The weighted age-specific rates are summed to produce the directly standardized rate. Again, this is simply a weighted average of the county-specific mortality rates based on the proportion of people in the U.S. population. We can repeat this process for any county to obtain comparable rates across counties.

We use the superscript T to refer to the target population (e.g., Elder County) and the superscript S to indicate the standard population (e.g., the United States). Recall also that the symbol Σ indicates that we are summing over all values right of the symbol. The notation $\sum \text{population size}_i^S$, for example, shows that we are summing over the population within age stratum i within the standard population S to obtain the total population size.

In the context of our Elder County example, we can express this notation as follows:

$$\text{Directly Standardized Rate} = \sum_{i=1}^{n}\left[\frac{\text{death count in elder county}_i}{\text{residents in elder county}_i} \times \frac{\text{US population}_i}{\sum \text{US population}_i} \right]$$

If we examine the calculation where i equals "old age", the calculations would be applied as follows (see Table 8.2):

$$\frac{\text{death count in elder county}_{\text{Old Age}}}{\text{population in elder county}_{\text{Old Age}}} \times \frac{\text{US population}_{\text{Old Age}}}{\text{US population}_{\text{All Ages}}}$$

$$0.01324309 = 0.047 \times 0.28177 = \frac{1,840}{39,142} \times \frac{50,992,996}{180,975,143}$$

We can repeat this for each age group to obtain the group-specific values. The sum of those group-specific values produces our directly standardized death rate for Elder County.

Directly Standardized Death Rate for Elder County: *0.01513* = 0.00106464 + 0.00063076 + 0.00106464 + 0.01324309

The age-adjusted, or directly standardized, mortality rate for Elder County is 15.1 deaths per 1,000—a considerable difference from the crude rate of 19.7 deaths per 1,000 (not adjusting for age). Not only is the standardized death rate considerably lower than the crude rate that we were so alarmed about at the beginning of this chapter, but the adjusted rate is actually lower than the national rate! That is, once we account for the age distribution of the evaluated group, the mortality rate is lower than that of the national population!

Okay, Mike, enough chit-chat. Show me how to do this in code. Certainly. An example calculation in Python is shown as follows:

```
population_US = [43327382, 45660395, 40994370, 50992996]
proportion_US = [0.23941, 0.25230, 0.22652, 0.28177]
population_Elder = [6524, 8698, 10148, 39142]
deaths_Elder = [5, 22, 48, 1840]

standard_population = sum(population_US)
adjusted_rate = 0

for i in range(len(population_Elder)):
    adjusted_rate += (deaths_Elder[i] / population_
Elder[i]) * (population_US[i] / standard_population)

directly_standardized_death_rate = adjusted_rate

print("Directly Standardized Death Rate for Elder
County:", directly_standardized_death_rate)
```

Nothing magical is happening in this code, and we are not relying on any specific Python libraries. It's worth mentioning that generally, when we see the summation symbol Σ in notation, it means that some iteration is needed in the code. In the Python code above, we iterate by looping over each age group *i* using a simple for loop. Note also that the += operator is shorthand to indicate that the value on the right-hand side should be added to the existing value stored within the variable on the left-hand side.

Staying true to the vectorized nature of the R, we can implement directly standardized rates in R:

```
population_US <- c(43327382, 45660395, 40994370,
50992996)
proportion_US <- c(0.23941, 0.25230, 0.22652, 0.28177)
population_Elder <- c(6524, 8698, 10148, 39142)
deaths_Elder <- c(5, 22, 48, 1840)

standard_population <- sum(population_US)

adjusted_rate <- sum((deaths_Elder / population_Elder) *
(population_US / standard_population))

cat("Directly Standardized Death Rate for Elder County:",
adjusted_rate, "\n")
```

Indirect Standardization

Of all the techniques in this book, I would venture to say that I use indirect standardization the most often. It is an incredibly versatile tool that can be applied to a wide range of healthcare research problems. While it is most often used to fairly compare health outcomes and disease frequency across groups with differing populations, like direct standardization, it can be used to standardize any metric, especially when the distribution of characteristics for the observations in the analysis can affect our expectation of an event or outcome. Perhaps we are interested in knowing if PPE supplies within a hospital are more or less than expected given the unique characteristics of the hospital and its patient mix (e.g., teaching hospital, urban/rural status, case mix index). We might be interested in knowing if the incidence of readmissions is more or less than expected, given the clinical and demographic characteristics of the evaluated patient population. An example in my research is the evaluation of ICD coding intensity and specificity, where our research team used indirect standardization to determine if hospitals were sufficiently recording diagnosis and procedure codes at the appropriate breadth and depth (while controlling for patient and hospital characteristics). Indirect standardization allows the researcher to control for various factors in a population to improve fairness in comparing event frequency.

How is this different from direct standardization, Mike? In direct standardization, we adjusted the group rates based on the proportion of individuals within the standard population within an age stratum—that is, we are adjusting the group rate to be comparable with the rate of the standard population. Indirect standardization, on the other hand, compares the actual observed events (e.g., deaths) with an expectation of the event that is adjusted based on our knowledge of the standard population.

Typically, with this method, the indirectly standardized values are expressed as a ratio of what actually happened (the observed events) to what we would have expected to happen, given what we know about the standard population (the expected events). An indirectly standardized ratio can be expressed as follows:

$$\text{indirectly standardized ratio} = \frac{O^T}{E^T} = \frac{\text{what actually happened}}{\text{what we expected to happen}}$$

An O/E ratio greater than 1 indicates that the number of observed events is higher than what we would expect of the target population. Conversely, an O/E less than 1 denotes fewer cases than expected, given the composition of the target population. In the context of mortality or care complications, the O/E ratio is sometimes called the SMR, which stands for "standard mortality ratio" or "standard morbidity ratio".

Some researchers prefer to convert the indirectly standardized ratio to a risk-standardized rate, a more interpretable metric. To obtain a risk-standardized rate, we must know the crude rate of the standard population.

$$\text{crude reference rate} = \frac{\text{event count}^S}{\text{population size}^S}$$

In our working example, the crude reference rate would be the national death rate. The indirectly standardized rate can be obtained by multiplying the O/E times the crude reference rate.

$$\text{Indirectly standardized rate for}$$
$$\text{the target population} = \frac{O^T}{E^T} \times \text{crude reference rate}$$

I like to think of this as using the O/E ratio to adjust the crude rate, where an O/E greater than 1 adjusts up the crude rate up, and an O/E less than 1 adjusts down the crude rate. The result is the standardized rate that can be compared across groups or target populations.

The indirectly standardized rate is analogous to a directly standardized rate; however, indirect standardization provides greater flexibility. We can evaluate the aggregated observed events relative to the expected events in their raw form, as a ratio, or as a difference. Others will argue that direct standardization is a more direct and interpretable approach and will prefer this approach over indirect standardization (Table 8.3).

An example will prove helpful here. Using the data from Elder County (target population) once again and our knowledge of U.S. (standard population) death rates, we can produce an expected number of deaths for each age

TABLE 8.3

An Example of Direct Standardization of Elder County Mortality Rates

Age Range Description	Age Range	Standard Population Death Rate (U.S.)	Target Population Population (Elder)	Observed Deaths (Elder)	Expected Deaths (Elder)
Young Adult	18–25	0.00087	6,524	5	6
Adult	26–44	0.00251	8,698	21	22
Middle Age	45–59	0.00483	10,148	47	49
Old Age	60+	0.052	39,142	1,839	2,035
Total			64,512	1,912	2,112

stratum. The expected deaths are calculated by multiplying the proportion of deaths in the U.S. population by the age-specific population within Elder County. In other words, we are saying, how many deaths would we expect from this age group in Elder County if the death rate was the same as the national population? Those observed deaths are subsequently used within a ratio of observed to expected events, such that ratio values greater than 1 indicate more deaths than expected, while ratios less than one indicate fewer deaths than expected.

One benefit of this approach is that the observed and expected values can be summed across age groups to obtain ratios at different levels of aggregation. For example, we might sum the observed and expected deaths across the middle and old age groups to produce an overall ratio of observed to expected deaths specific to the combination of those two age groups.

The formula for indirect standardization would take the following form:

$$E^T = \text{expected events}^T = \sum_{i=1}^{n} \left[\text{population size}_i^T \times \frac{\text{event count}_i^S}{\Sigma \text{event count}_i^S} \right]$$

Again, this notation shows how the proportion of deaths $\frac{\text{event count}_i^S}{\Sigma \text{event count}_i^S}$ in the standard population S for age group i is multiplied by the population of the population size for the target population T to obtain the expected number of events for age stratum i. We use the large sigma operator to sum over age-specific expected values to obtain the total expected values for the target population. Total observed events are simply the summation of events for the target population T across age strata i.

$$O^T = \text{observed events} = \sum_{i=1}^{n} \text{event count}_i^T$$

The result is the indirectly standardized ratio for the target population $\dfrac{O^T}{E^T}$, which can again be converted to an indirectly standardized rate by multiplying the O/E by the crude reference rate:

$$\text{Indirectly standardized rate} = \frac{O^T}{E^T} \times \text{crude reference rate}$$

Or, in the context of our Elder County example, the calculation would be as follows:

$$\text{Indirectly standardized ratio for the target population} = 0.905 = \frac{1,912}{2,112}$$
$$= \frac{O^{\text{Elder}}}{E^{\text{Elder}}}$$

The national death rate in our dataset is $0.0166 = \dfrac{3,004,187}{180,975,143}$ (or 16.6 deaths per 1,000), which allows us to obtain an indirectly standardized rate for Elder County as follows:

$$\text{Indirectly standardized rate for the Elder County} = 0.015 = \frac{1,912}{2,112} \times .016$$

O/E ratios can be informative, allowing comparability across groups regardless of magnitude. For example, an O/E ratio of 2 might computed from a ratio of 2,000/1,000 or 20,000/10,000. One drawback with ratios, however, is that they can mask important information contained in the expected value, especially when 0 events occur. Imagine counties A and B have 0 deaths; however, through indirect standardization, county A's O/E ratio is 0/10, and county B's is 0/1,000. While counties A and B have an O/E of 0 using this method, county B's mortality is arguably significantly lower than expected. Several strategies can be employed to mitigate this issue (e.g., shrinkage estimators), although these methods are more advanced and are outside of the scope of this book.

But Mike, this method only controls for a single variable like age, right? What if I want to control for multiple factors? Great question. Indirect standardization can be implemented in various ways to control for multiple variables. Perhaps we wanted to control for a person's age and sex to produce a more precise expected value (since death rates by age differ by sex). Intuitively, the most direct way to control for multiple characteristics would be to create more specific strata. We would have a female *and* male stratum for each age group, doubling the strata used to produce the expected values. This is perfectly acceptable; however, we quickly encounter the *curse of dimensionality* as we add additional control variables. Imagine adding other population characteristics, such as income and health insurance coverage. Each additional control variable exponentially increases the number of strata, with each stratum representing a narrower population subset. As you might imagine, this approach becomes problematic when conducting robust analyses where the research question requires controlling for a wide range of personal characteristics.

A more elegant alternative is to use regression or other predictive models to produce an expected value for each observation (or person) in our analysis. Using this approach, we would regress the event (as the response variable) on a set of person characteristics (predictors) to obtain an expected event. Rather than using strata from the standard population to produce a (crude) expectation of risk, the regression approach would allow us to generalize the data in the standard population through a fitted model. In our mortality example, we would regress the binary indicator of mortality on a broad set of person characteristics to obtain the probability of mortality. This probability may serve as the expected value for a given individual. We can then sum over all the probabilities produced through the regression model to obtain the total expected events for the target population.

The formula for our logistic regression might look like this:

$$Y_{ijk} \sim \text{Ber}(P_i)$$

and

$$\log\left(\frac{P_i}{1-P_i}\right) = \alpha + \beta_1(\text{age}_i) + \beta_2(\text{sex}_i) + \beta_3(\text{disease group}_i)$$

Recall that logistic regression is a GLM that models the log odds of an outcome through its linear combination of predictors. To obtain the probability, we use the sigmoid function as the inverse link function to produce the probability of an event.

$$P_i = \frac{1}{1 + e^{-\alpha + \beta_1(\text{age}_i) + \beta_2(\text{sex}_i) + \beta_3(\text{disease group}_i)}}$$

This probability *p* will serve as an expected value in the context of standardization of a binary outcome.

When using regression modeling for indirect standardization, the model is typically fit using the data of the standard population and applied to the target population. In this way, the expected values from the model represent what we would expect of the larger general population, providing the same distribution of characteristics of the target population.

Table 8.4 includes 25 mock high-risk individuals with an indicator of death (observed) and a probability of death (expected). The expected value results from applying a logistic regression model (fit based on the standard population) to the target population.

As shown in Table 8.4, we can sum over the observed and expected values to obtain an indirectly standardized ratio:

$$\text{indirectly standardized ratio} = 0.822 = \frac{9}{10.9433} = \frac{O^T}{E^T}$$

TABLE 8.4

Sample Observed and Expected Values Aggregated to Produce a Ratio of Observed to Expected Events

Person	Observed	Expected
1	1	0.4200
2	0	0.0008
3	0	0.0430
4	0	0.2700
5	0	0.0001
6	1	0.8500
7	0	0.0000
8	1	0.8499
9	1	0.8006
10	0	0.3679
11	1	0.8506
12	0	0.1772
13	1	0.7498
14	0	0.3527
15	0	0.5160
16	0	0.3652
17	0	0.1042
18	1	0.8970
19	0	0.1240
20	0	0.0001
21	0	0.7839
22	0	0.3860
23	1	0.7907
24	1	0.8987
25	0	0.3450
Total	9	10.9433

Expected values for other events (e.g., income) can also be calculated using the appropriate statistical model. For income estimation, we might choose a zero-inflated model (some individuals are unemployed) or a Poisson regression. Expected values are simply the best estimate of the event based on the patient characters used in the model.

In population studies, we often do not have the data at the individual level to indirectly standardize the data in this way, but when it is available, the method comes with many benefits. A person-level expected value (while often not reliable on its own) can be aggregated to different levels to form indirectly standardized ratios at different. Perhaps we want to know if Elder County, FL, has a higher standardized death rate than Millennial County, CA. A person-level model will allow us to adjust for the many person-level factors that cause those populations to differ to obtain a comparable mortality rate. We could further aggregate to lower levels of aggregation such as census tract.

Indirectly standardizing the data further allows mortality rates to be measured over time simply by grouping the evaluated population into temporal units (day, week, month, etc.).

Let's look at a reproducible example in Python. As shown below, there are two steps for indirect standardization: (1) fitting a model based on the standard population and (2) applying the fitted model to a target population to produce the expected values. The observed and expected values from the target population are summed to form the observed to expected, or O/E, ratio.

```python
import numpy as np
import pandas as pd
import statsmodels.api as sm

np.random.seed(42)
n = 1000

age = np.random.randint(18, 90, n)
sex = np.random.choice(['Male', 'Female'], n)
ms_drg = np.random.choice(['DRG1', 'DRG2', 'DRG3'], n)
mortality = np.random.choice([0, 1], n)

standard_data = pd.DataFrame({'Age': age, 'Sex': sex,
'MS-DRG': ms_drg, 'Mortality': mortality})

print(standard_data)

standard_X = pd.get_dummies(standard_data[['Age', 'Sex',
'MS-DRG']], drop_first=True, dtype=int)
standard_y = standard_data['Mortality']

standard_X = sm.add_constant(standard_X)

logit_model = sm.Logit(standard_y, standard_X)
standard_model = logit_model.fit()
```

```
target_n = 200
target_data = pd.DataFrame({
    'Age': np.random.randint(18, 90, target_n),
    'Sex': np.random.choice(['Male', 'Female'],
target_n),
    'MS-DRG': np.random.choice(['DRG1', 'DRG2', 'DRG3'],
target_n)
})

target_X = pd.get_dummies(target_data[['Age', 'Sex',
'MS-DRG']], drop_first=True, dtype=int)
target_X = sm.add_constant(target_X)

predicted_prob = standard_model.predict(target_X)

target_data['Mortality'] = np.random.choice([0, 1],
target_n)

expected_events = predicted_prob.sum()

observed_events = target_data['Mortality'].sum()
observed_to_expected_ratio = observed_events /
expected_events

print(f"Observed events: {observed_events}")
print(f"Expected events: {expected_events}")
print(f"Observed to Expected Ratio:
{observed_to_expected_ratio}")
```

Similarly in R, there are two steps—fitting the model and applying the model to produce the expected values—the sum of which serve as the denominator of our risk adjusted ratio.

```
set.seed(42)

n <- 1000

age <- sample(18:89, n, replace = TRUE)
sex <- sample(c('Male', 'Female'), n, replace = TRUE)
ms_drg <- sample(c('DRG1', 'DRG2', 'DRG3'), n, replace =
TRUE)
mortality <- sample(c(0, 1), n, replace = TRUE)

standard_data <- data.frame(Age = age, Sex = sex, MS_DRG
= ms_drg, Mortality = mortality)

print(standard_data)

standard_data$Sex <- as.factor(standard_data$Sex)
standard_data$MS_DRG <- as.factor(standard_data$MS_DRG)

logit_model <- glm(Mortality ~ Age + Sex + MS_DRG, data =
standard_data, family = binomial)
```

```
target_n <- 200
target_data <- data.frame(
   Age = sample(18:89, target_n, replace = TRUE),
   Sex = sample(c('Male', 'Female'), target_n, replace =
TRUE),
   MS_DRG = sample(c('DRG1', 'DRG2', 'DRG3'), target_n,
replace = TRUE),
   mortality = sample(c(0, 1), target_n, replace = TRUE)
)

target_data$Sex <- as.factor(target_data$Sex)
target_data$MS_DRG <- as.factor(target_data$MS_DRG)

predicted_prob <- predict(logit_model, newdata = target_
data, type = "response")
expected_events <- sum(predicted_prob)

observed_events <- sum(target_data$mortality)
observed_to_expected_ratio <- observed_events /
expected_events

cat("Observed events:", observed_events, "\n")
cat("Expected events:", expected_events, "\n")
cat("Observed to Expected Ratio:", observed_to_expected_
ratio, "\n")
```

Risk Adjustment

Risk adjustment is a special form of indirect standardization used to measure variation in quality and efficiency across care settings. With risk adjustment, our goal is not simply to standardize the rates but to identify opportunities to improve quality of care and utilization. Health plans, such as Medicare Advantage, also use risk models to assess patients' health statuses and predict their healthcare needs, which helps determine fair and accurate payments to providers based on the complexity and severity of the patient population they serve. If you read Chapter 2 on healthcare measures (no judgment if you didn't), we discussed several sets of healthcare measures that use risk adjustment to compare the observed outcome of care to an expectation given the unique clinical and demographic characteristics of the patient population. These measures include the AHRQ patient safety indicators, NHSN healthcare-associated infections, Yale CORE outcome measures (e.g., mortality, readmissions, complications), and CMS Medicare Spending Per Beneficiary measure. Risk adjustment is the gold standard for quality and efficiency measurement, and any credible evaluation of quality and efficiency uses some form of risk adjustment to ensure that the variation in care controls the patient mix.

Risk adjustment models are typically fit based on national population (or nationally representative) and applied to patients within some sub-population, such as a health system, hospital, physician, or service line. The expected value in the context of risk adjustment is an estimate of the outcome if the patient received the generalized care of the standard population. If we observed a greater number of outcomes than expected, controlling for the range of patient characteristics, we make the assumption that the difference in observed and expected outcomes is a result of patient care.

In the risk modeling process, it is important to distinguish pre-existing patient conditions from those arising during hospitalization. This is a critical distinction, as including conditions resulting from care can mask important variation in patient outcomes.

Let's look at an exaggerated example to illustrate. You've developed two risk models designed to produce an expected length of stay for a patient's hospitalization. These models were fit using the National Inpatient Sample (NIS) dataset from Healthcare Cost and Utilization Project (HCUP) as the standard population. We want to use this risk model to evaluate the variation in length of stay on a med/surg unit at Elder Memorial, a new short-term care hospital in the region.

The length of stay risk models will be used to compare the total observed days to the total expected days in the form of an O/E, with observed and expected totals simply being the summation of patient days across all patient hospitalizations. In the case of total expected days, we simply sum the predicted values from of our regression model to obtain the total expected days.

The first risk model includes a curated set of risk factors, including patient age, sex, and a set of chronic conditions (e.g., cancer, diabetes, heart disease, stroke). Again, the standard population was used to fit this model, regressing the length of stay on this set of patient characteristics.

The second model, a data-driven model, incorporates a broader set of clinical variables using diagnosis and procedure codes available within the standard dataset. The second model is a better fit with improved mean squared error and a higher r-squared value.

Not only does this second model identify a broader set of variables that explain variation in length of stay, the O/E values for Elder Memorial are much better! Why would we not use the more complete and better-fit second model?

You approach the chief medical officer at Elder Memorial for input on which model should be employed—making a compelling case for the second model. In reviewing the patient characteristics used in the model, she points out that complications of care, such as pressure ulcers, falls, and infections, are included as predictors in the model. Here, we have broken the fundamental rule of risk adjustment in that the model should not control for the care received by the provider, as it can mask important variation in quality.

By including these complications of care, we would expect longer lengths of stay for patients experiencing complications, thereby masking a quality-of-care problem! The favorable O/E values in the second (poorly designed) model essentially factors out suboptimal care by including complications of care as predictors.

Despite the better fit of the second model, the first model is the proper choice, as the increased error in the model fit exposes true care variation through the O/E ratio.

Risk adjustment is not about extreme optimization, but rather properly controlling, to the best extent possible, for the range of patient clinical and demographic that might affect a patient's outcome, such that differences between observed and expected events exposes gaps in care.

Present on Admission (POA) Status

How do we distinguish between preexisting patient clinical conditions and those developing during the care process within administrative data? If you recall from Chapter 1, patient diagnoses are accompanied by a present-on-admission indicator (POA) that informs us if the condition was preexisting or developed in the hospital. We could examine COVID-19, for example. A patient might present with COVID-19 upon admission, or COVID-19 may be hospital-acquired—that is, the patient acquired COVID-19 due to improper hand washing, cleanliness, etc.

When developing a risk model, it is important to narrow the risk factors to those present on admission. This prevents us from lowering the bar for suboptimal care (i.e., unduly inflating the expected value).

Race and Ethnicity

It is important to note that race and ethnicity (standard variables available in administrative data) as social constructs should not be used within risk adjustment models, as we would not want to change our expectation of an outcome simply due to a patient's racial identification. Imagine if a particular racial group was highly associated with an adverse outcome. Controlling for race in our risk model would produce a higher expectation of the outcome for that racial group, thereby masking important variation in care that may be informative from a health equity perspective. We should not expect a patient to have better or worse outcomes simply due to racial identity.

While this is a general rule, there are rare exceptions where there is clinical standing for including race and ethnicity, such as the evaluation of sickle cell anemia in black patients. If race and ethnicity are included in a risk model, the measure developer should ensure rigorous clinical justification grounded in the scientific literature.

We are often interested in understanding inequities in care across different racial and ethnic groups, however, and a helpful technique is *stratification*, where the risk-adjusted results (i.e., the O/E values) are segmented across demographic groups. In this case, the goal is to surface potential disparities in care from the differing O/E ratios across strata.

Social Drivers of Health

An important topic being discussed in the healthcare literature is that of social drivers of health (SDoHs) and health outcomes, and naturally, there are conversations among experts about how to incorporate such variables in risk adjustment models. To help guide this conversation, an important distinction should be made between risk models solely designed to improve quality and efficiency and those that tie performance to reputation, reward, and reimbursement.

Let us say that your patient dataset also includes a patient-level SDoH index variable—a composite value comprised of income, food insecurity, access to transportation, disability, etc. There is uncertainty on whether this index should be used as a control variable in the risk model.

If the goal is to measure true quality and efficiency of care, variables related to SDoH should not be included. As with race and ethnicity, we do not want to lower the bar for a patient population serving more marginalized patients by controlling for SDoH. In this way, variation can be surfaced and acted upon by the hospital and the larger community. Again, stratification as a secondary step can be a valuable tool to identify quality and efficiency disparities across SDoH factors.

If we shift the scenario to risk models used to determine a hospital or physician's reputation (e.g., CMS Overall Star Rating) or reimbursement (e.g., Hospital Value-Based Purchasing, MIPS), we must change our perspective. Studies have shown that hospitals serving more historically marginalized populations generally have worse outcomes (even when controlling for clinical and demographic characteristics). Hospitals serving such populations should not be penalized simply due to the populations they serve. In these scenarios, it is necessary to control for SDoH so that hospitals providing high-quality care to those more marginalized patient populations can still be recognized for high quality and avoid penalties for variation in care outside of their control.

Stratification

In the indirect standardization example from the previous section, the patient's disease group (AMI, heart failure, pneumonia, stroke, CABG, etc.) was controlled for using MS-DRG. While this might be sufficient in some scenarios, it is necessary to consider how the effect of the remaining patient characteristics on outcomes might change within the context of a disease group. Imagine that our risk adjustment model is evaluating the binary occurrence of a complication for hospital stays—a standard metric within healthcare quality measurement. Intuitively, a patient's risk of a complication will increase as age increases. However, if we evaluate the association between age and complications across specific disease strata, we might see considerably different associations depending on the disease stratum evaluated. The point here is that the relationship between a patient's risk factors, and an outcome will vary within the context of a disease stratum—a data concern that cannot be resolved by simply adding a disease group variable in the regression model. Remember that regression models assume that each predictor variable (or risk factor) is independent, and including a disease group variable will not mitigate this issue.

As such, for some risk adjustment models, it is worth considering stratifying models by disease group (i.e., fitting a separate model for each group) so that the unique relationship between patient factors and outcomes can be modeled in a more clinically appropriate manner. While the implementation requires separate models to be developed for each outcome, the end result will be a more clinically relevant risk estimation. Of course, some machine learning models, such as tree- and neural network-based models, will naturally account for the complex interaction between variables (i.e., features) and are not bound to the assumptions of independence.

It should be noted that the resulting expected values can be aggregated across disease group strata. Even if our risk model has 500 disease strata (with a regression model specific to each disease stratum). The observed and expected values from those stratum-specific models can still be aggregated to form an overall observed-to-expected ratio (while adjusting for disease/covariate interaction as stated above).

Coding Variation

Recall from Chapter 2 that measures using administrative data can be sensitive to variability in coding rigor, which includes the intensity (i.e., breadth) and specificity (i.e., depth of coding). Providers with more rigorous coding practices will identify more risk in the patient population, which can inflate the number of expected cases, resulting in a lower O/E value. Some measure developers will attempt to control for variation in coding risk through coding indices that quantify variation in coding.

Re-baselining

Risk adjustment models must be maintained (or re-fit) at routine intervals so that the generalized information about the standard population reflects the most current practices of care, distributions of patient characteristics, and the resulting expectation of an event. This process of refitting the risk model is referred to as "re-baselining" or "recalibration". The COVID-19 pandemic is a prime (although extreme) example of how the distribution of patient characteristics and the outcome prevalence can change over time. If the standard population is wildly different from the target population that we wish to standardize, our estimates may over or underestimate that population's risk. Failure to re-baseline the risk model at regular intervals (e.g., annually) can lead to suboptimal risk estimations.

Another reason to rebaseline risk models developed using administrative data is to ensure that the fitted model incorporates the most recent coding standards. The ICD-10 coding system and the resulting MS-DRGs are now updated biannually. This means that new ICD-10 and MS-DRG codes can be introduced every six months, and others can be discontinued. Other coding systems, such as the CCSR and HCC disease grouping, are also subject to change. Therefore, if the risk model is fit against a standard population from a time period before such coding changes, the risk associated with newly-introduced codes will go undetected in the more current target population. This was the case with the introduction of the COVID-19 ICD-10 code, as previous risk models did not have knowledge of the COVID-19 code and could not detect the critical risk associated with this disease.

The Importance of Peer Groups in Risk Adjustment

While risk models are an important tool for comparing variation in quality, efficiency, and patient complexity across entities with differing risk profiles (i.e., different distribution of patient characteristics), studies have shown that risk models can only control for differing characteristics within limits.

An urban level I trauma center will have a significantly different patient population than a small rural hospital. Even with risk-adjusted O/E values, we would not want to compare the performance of the large urban hospital to the small rural hospital. That is, we cannot assume that the performance level of one hospital with its unique case mix is obtainable from another hospital with a notably different case mix.

This is especially important when setting goals using risk-adjusted results. Healthcare entities often compare their risk-adjusted performance against a higher-performing peer group (e.g., the top-performing decile). Without considering the hospital's structural characteristics (through peer groups or other methods), we might set unreasonable performance expectations.

Therefore, it is helpful to evaluate risk-adjusted results, or O/E values, within a group of comparable facilities. This allows healthcare entities to assess their risk-adjusted results in the context of a comparable set of facilities.

Statistical Significance and Confidence Intervals

Previously, we discussed how confidence intervals for means, proportions, odds ratios, and regression coefficients can be calculated. A risk-adjusted ratio (or indirectly standardized ratio) of observed to expected events will also have some degree of sampling error. While quantifying the degree of uncertainty of an O/E ratio is incredibly useful, experts debate how to best identify such error.

Given that this is a book designed for beginners, I'll share one of the more frequently employed methods for calculating confidence intervals for risk standardized ratios; however, the reader should know that more advanced statisticians and epidemiologists will have their own justification for using alternative methods.

Byar's Approximation

Many methods to calculate confidence intervals for an O/E ratio will calculate the error of the observed value, holding the expected value as fixed. This is one criticism of these methods, in that they assume that there is only sampling error in the distribution of observed events, ignoring the inherent error from the model fit of the regression model that produced the expected values. Setting this criticism aside for now, the confidence interval of a risk-adjusted ratio can be expressed as follows:

$$\frac{O^{\text{Lower}}}{E} < \frac{O}{E} < \frac{O^{\text{Upper}}}{E}$$

The name of the method discussed in this chapter is Byar's approximation—a technique that is easily implemented without complex iteration required of more precise (or "exact") methods. Recall that binary variables summed to some level of aggregation (e.g., hospital, physician, service line) result in a count of events and that count data typically follows a Poisson distribution—characterized by its rightward skew (or more formally, the mean is equal to the variance). Therefore, these approximation methods quantify error by assuming that the observed counts follow a Poisson distribution.

The formulas for the Byar's approximation are given below, showing how the lower and upper confidence intervals are calculated. We can adjust the confidence level as needed through the z-value $z_{a/2}$ (e.g., ~1.96 for a 95% CI). As discussed in Chapter 3, α refers to the significance level (e.g., $\alpha = .05$ for a 95% confidence level). Since we are interested in the error on both ends of the distribution, we use $\alpha/2$ to indicate that the 5% Type I error probability is split to each end of the distribution (i.e., .025 on each end).

The theoretical underpinnings of this approach are outside of the scope of this book. The implementation, however, is relatively simple (relative to other approaches) and is shown below:

$$O^{\text{Lower}} = O \times \left(1 - \frac{1}{9O} - \frac{z_{a/2}}{3} \times \sqrt{\frac{1}{O}} \right)^3$$

$$O^{\text{Upper}} = (O+1) \times \left(1 - \frac{1}{9(O+1)} - \frac{z_{a/2}}{3} \times \sqrt{\frac{1}{O+1}} \right)^3$$

$$\frac{O^{\text{Lower}}}{E} < \frac{O}{E} < \frac{O^{\text{Upper}}}{E}$$

At the time of this book, there is no popularized library for calculating confidence intervals for standardized ratios (including Byar's approximation), so the Python code below is a conversion of an excerpt from the epi.smr function found in the R epiR package. epiR is a time-tested library regularly used for this purpose maintained by the University of Melbourne, Australia. I suspect these methods will soon be incorporated into statsmodels (or another well-supported statistical library) in Python.

```
import numpy as np
from scipy.stats import norm
def smr_byar_approx(obs=4, exp=3.3, conf_level=0.95):
```

```
    if isinstance(obs, list) or isinstance(exp, list):
        raise ValueError("Arguments obs and exp must be
of length 1")

    N = 1 - ((1 - conf_level) / 2)
    z = norm.ppf(N, loc=0, scale=1)

    a = obs
    lambda_ = exp
    smr = a / lambda_

    if a % int(a) != 0:
        raise ValueError("Argument obs must be a whole
number")

    # Byar's approximation:
    if a < lambda_:
        _a = a + 1
    else:
        _a = a

    byar_z = ((9 * _a) ** 0.5) * (1 - (1 / (9 * _a)) -
((lambda_ / _a) ** (1 / 3)))
    byar_p = 2 * norm.cdf(byar_z, loc=0, scale=1)
if byar_z < 0 else 2 * (1 - norm.cdf(byar_z, loc=0,
scale=1))

    # Confidence interval - Regidor et al. (1993):
    alow = a * (1 - (1 / (9 * a)) - (z / 3) * np.sqrt(1 /
a)) ** 3
    aupp = (a + 1) * (1 - (1 / (9 * (a + 1))) + (z / 3) *
np.sqrt(1 / (a + 1))) ** 3

    byar_low = alow / lambda_
    byar_upp = aupp / lambda_

    rval = {
        'obs': a,
        'exp': lambda_,
        'est': smr,
        'lower': byar_low,
        'upper': byar_upp,
        'test_statistic': byar_z,
        'p_value': byar_p
    }
    return rval
```

In R, we have the convenience of using the epiR package:

```
library(epiR)
obs <- 4
```

```
exp <- 3.3
result <- epi.smr(obs, exp, conf.level = .95) #Byar is
the default method
print(result)
```

The method (shown in Python and R) produces the upper and lower confidence intervals, test statistic, and *p*-value, as well as the calculated observed and expected values and resulting O/E ratio (or SMR).

We discussed these components in detail in Chapter 4. Please see the section on Confidence Intervals if you've skipped that chapter (or fell asleep).

The main benefit of confidence intervals, like those used for means and proportions, is that with smaller samples, there is a greater degree of sampling error. Byar's approximation and comparable methods will widen the confidence interval with smaller samples and narrow it with larger samples.

It should be noted that Byar's approximation is accurate even with small numbers; however, more precise methods are generally preferred when the observed event count is five or less. In these cases, a more sophisticated but more accurate estimation can be obtained using the mid-P exact method (which is outside of the scope of this book)

One question that might arise is why we can't use one of the hypothesis tests in Chapter 3 to compare observed to expected events. For example, if we know the observed and expected counts of events, can we not simply use a z-test or t-test to compare the two distributions and determine statistical significance and confidence intervals?

In short, we can use standard hypothesis testing, but it is important to know that we are violating some of the assumptions of the statistical tests. The difficulty is that the observed and expected values are Non-IID", which stands for "non-independent and identically distributed". Let's break this down a bit more:

Outcomes that are *non-independent* imply that the observations or data points being evaluated are not independent of each other. In an IID scenario, each data point is assumed to be unrelated to the others. However, in non-independent data, the value of one observation might be related to or influenced by other observations. For instance, in time series data, each data point might depend on previous data points, violating the independence assumption. For our example, as it relates to comparing observed to expected values, this is not the driving concern.

The second "I" refers to *non-identically distributed* data. In an IID scenario, it's assumed that each data point comes from the same probability distribution. In our example, the observed distribution is of a different type than the expected distribution. For example, if we evaluate observed and expected events at the patient level, the observed events follow a Bernoulli distribution (yes or no), and the expected events are probabilities. The same is true, although less impactful, is the comparison of count data from an observed distribution (e.g., LOS) with that of a continuous expected distribution.

The foremost expert on risk adjustment modeling, Lisa Iezzoni, proposes an approach (among others) to identify statistically significant deviations between observed and expected events using traditional one sample z- and t-tests despite the IID assumption being violated. A reference to some of Iezzoni's work is provided at the end of this chapter. I strongly recommend her excellent work to anyone serious about building robust risk adjustment models.

For brevity however, we've focused on Byar's approximation in this chapter, as it does not violate IID assumptions and is often used to compare indirectly standardized ratios; however, the reader is encouraged to explore the other methods proposed by Iezzoni and others.

Conclusion

You've reached the finish line once again (unless you skipped to the end—don't be that person). This chapter dives deep into two critical methods for comparing populations and understanding healthcare outcomes: direct and indirect standardization.

Direct standardization helps compare populations with different age distributions. It involves adjusting rates within a specific population to make them comparable to a standard population. This minimizes the influence of differing population structures, and ensures fairer comparisons.

Indirect standardization, my favorite technique, accomplishes a similar goal of comparing outcomes across groups with varied populations. Unlike direct standardization, it compares observed events with an expectation adjusted based on the standard population's knowledge. It uses ratios and predictive models, like logistic regression and other GLMs, to control for various population factors for a more accurate comparison.

We also touched on the important topic of risk adjustment in healthcare, which isn't just about standardizing rates but identifying gaps in care and utilization.

Additional Resources

Lash, T. L., VanderWeele, T. J., Haneuse, S., & Rothman, K. J. (2021). *Modern Epidemiology* (4th ed.). LWW.
Iezzoni, L. I. (2012). *Risk Adjustment for Measuring Health Care Outcomes* (4th ed.). Health Administration Press.

9

Time-to-Event Analysis

In this chapter, we will discuss *time-to-event* or *survival* analysis where the outcome of interest is the time to an event (e.g., days, months, years, until some outcome or event occurs) given some starting point (e.g., a cancer diagnosis). We might be interested in the number of days until remission (the event) from the date of a cancer diagnosis (starting point or "time origin"). We might also want to know if some exposure (e.g. treatment) affects the time until remission. While the terms time-to-event and survival analysis are interchangeable and refer to the same set of statistical methods, the applicability of these methods reaches far beyond evaluating survival in healthcare analyses. These methods may be used to measure the time until readmissions, complications, or onset of symptoms. They can also be used outside of the healthcare setting to assess customer churn, days until credit card default, species extinction, and related problems.

Now, you might be asking yourself: Why do we need special methods for these types of problems? Can we not use a regression-based approach to make inferences about a time to an event? Given that event times often have a rightward skewed distribution, we could certainly consider a GLM using an appropriate distribution, especially when we are interested in controlling for multiple confounders. In this scenario, we could just model the effect of some exposure (a predictor) on time (a response).

While these more traditional methods might be appropriate in some cases, the problem largely occurs when we have *censored* data in our dataset—observations for which the entire time duration is unknown within the study period.

Let's talk censoring. Figure 9.1 shows the event time from some time origin (e.g., a positive diagnosis of a condition) to an event (e.g., death) for a set of mock patients. The most common form of censoring is *right censoring*, which occurs when the event of interest (e.g. mortality) has yet to happen for a subject by the end of the study period or when they are *lost to follow-up*. We can see that the event time for some subjects extends beyond the study period, and as such, we lose sight of a potential incidence of an outcome (or event) past the study end date. These are the right censored subjects in the study. Loss to follow-up, a special type of right censoring, refers to subjects that

DOI: 10.1201/9781003609759-9

leave the study or can no longer be tracked. Here, too, we cannot know if an outcome occurred due to their unknown status.

Left censoring, a less common scenario, occurs when the event of interest occurs before the study start date and only the duration for a subject since the study start date is known. Examples of left censoring can be seen in Figure 9.1, where a subject's duration begins before the study period begins. We might know if the outcome occurred, but we do not know the entire duration of the event.

Interval censoring happens when an event occurs within the study period, but the exact event time is unknown. Perhaps a physician's office is following a patient through regular office visits, and an outcome occurs between visits. In this case, we know an event occurred within the study period, but we are unsure of the exact duration or event time. We only know that the time of an event falls between two observation time points. Interval censoring, like left censoring, is a less common scenario in time-to-event studies.

As a result, methods like regression are only suitable for censored data if they assume complete observation of outcomes. Time-to-event methods, on the other hand, are designed to gracefully handle censoring even when not all events are observed.

Another way to visualize event time is to align the duration for each subject based on the origin date (e.g. a cancer diagnosis). This interpretation of time, called *analysis time*, is shown in Figure 9.2 rather than linear time, shown in Figure 9.1. Arranging the observations in this way provides a better picture of survival up to a certain point within the time duration across subjects.

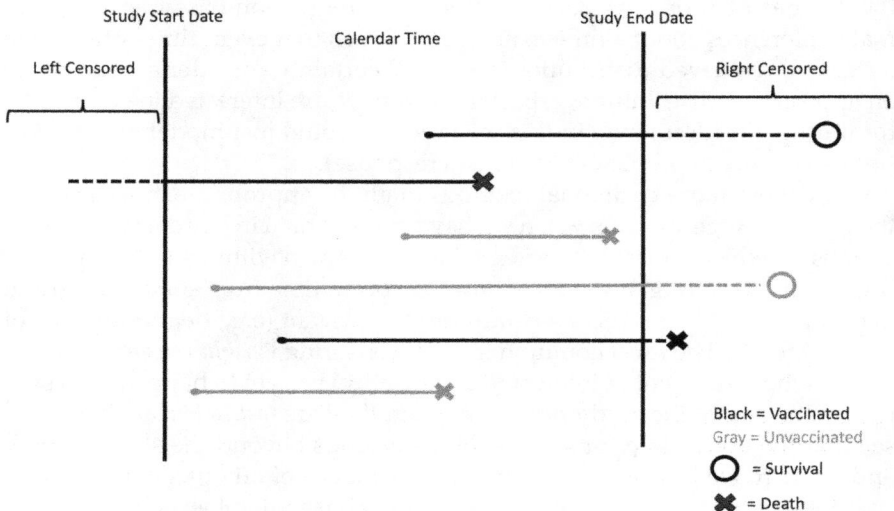

FIGURE 9.1
Examples of uncensored and left and right censored subjects over time.

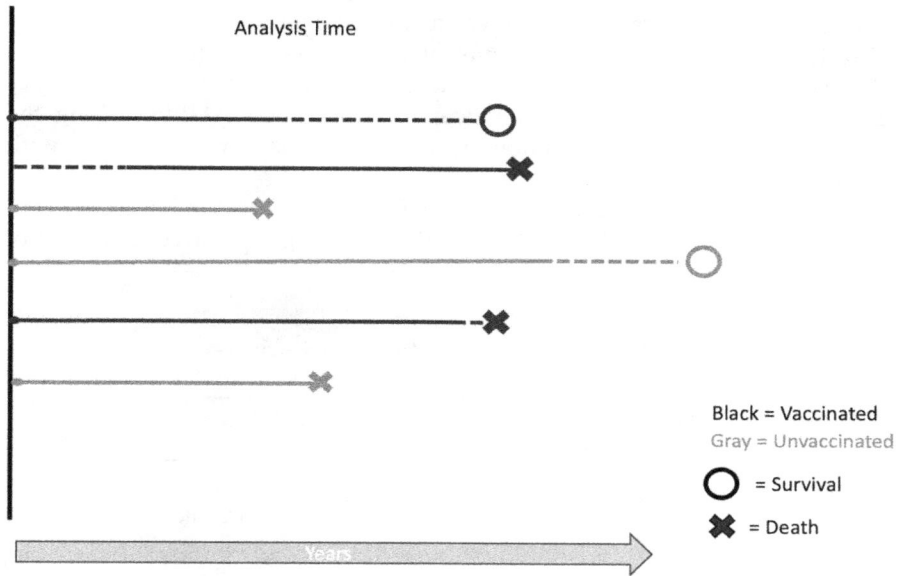

FIGURE 9.2

Examples of uncensored and left and right censored subjects aligned over analysis time.

When exploring time-to-event problems, analysts often rely on three key methods. First is the Kaplan–Meier curve, a useful visual representation of survival rates for one or more groups over time. The log-rank test, the second method, is a hypothesis test designed to test for the differences between survival curves. We might want to know, for example, if there is a statistically significant difference between the survival curves between two factors (treatment group A or B)—that is, do patients receiving treatment A generally survive longer than those receiving treatment B? Lastly, the Cox Proportional Hazards Regression, or Cox Regression, is a regression-based approach that helps researchers control for and quantify potential associations between multiple factors and survival probabilities.

The following sections will introduce these three methods; however, like all aspects of statistics, time-to-event analysis has many layers of depth. Additional resources have been provided at the end of this chapter for those interested in pursuing the subject further.

To keep it interesting (and I'm using the term "interesting" loosely), let's use a hypothetical scenario involving a rare disease. We'll call this disease Contagium-24 (or C-24).

C-24 is a rare genetic condition impacting the nervous system in adulthood, potentially resulting in paralysis and, in aggressive cases, mortality. Your research facility has been tracking survival for patients who elected to be vaccinated with an experimental therapeutic vaccine and those who have declined the vaccination. While not offering complete immunity to C24, this vaccine demonstrates the potential to considerably reduce the severity of the illness and its related symptoms. To assess its effectiveness, your lab has engaged in a decade-long study, monitoring patients from symptom onset and documenting instances of C24-related fatalities along the way. Specifically, we want to know if the C24 vaccination is associated with increased rates of survival.

The collected patient data is shown in Table 9.1. Here, we have the event time in years (with the start of the event time being a positive diagnosis of

TABLE 9.1

Includes Example Patients Diagnosed with C-25 Over a Ten-Year Study Period

Event Times (Years)	Age	Sex	Observed Event (Mortality)	Treatment Group
3	60	M	0	Vaccinated
3	48	F	0	Vaccinated
6	58	F	0	Vaccinated
4	74	M	1	Vaccinated
4	42	M	0	Vaccinated
3	64	M	0	Vaccinated
3	43	M	0	Vaccinated
5	26	F	0	Vaccinated
8	54	M	0	Vaccinated
8	59	M	1	Vaccinated
7	66	M	0	Vaccinated
6	55	F	1	Vaccinated
10	71	F	0	Vaccinated
4	43	F	0	Vaccinated
4	45	M	1	Vaccinated
4	46	M	1	Unvaccinated
4	35	M	1	Unvaccinated
4	34	F	0	Unvaccinated
9	54	M	1	Unvaccinated
7	45	M	0	Unvaccinated
3	60	U	1	Unvaccinated
3	69	M	0	Unvaccinated
6	41	M	1	Unvaccinated
6	74	F	1	Unvaccinated
7	46	F	0	Unvaccinated
4	85	F	1	Unvaccinated
4	60	M	1	Unvaccinated
2	66	M	1	Unvaccinated
7	67	F	1	Unvaccinated
5	73	M	1	Unvaccinated

C-24), along with the subject's age, sex, death indicator, and vaccination status. In time-to-event analysis, "censored" records are those where the event of interest (e.g., death, failure, recovery) hasn't occurred by the end of the study period or the time of data collection. Looking at the provided data, a "1" in the "Observed Event" column indicates an observed event (i.e., death), while a "0" indicates censored data, where the event has not occurred by the end of the study.

Now that we've prepared the data let's begin our analysis. We'll start with the Kaplan–Meier curve and log-rank test, complementary methods for comparing survival curves over time.

Kaplan–Meier Method

The Kaplan–Meier curve (Figure 9.3) is a graphical representation of survival or event occurrence over time. This non-parametric technique (i.e., we do not rely on specific assumptions about the underlying probability distributions) estimates the probability of an event happening at each time point, considering censored data.

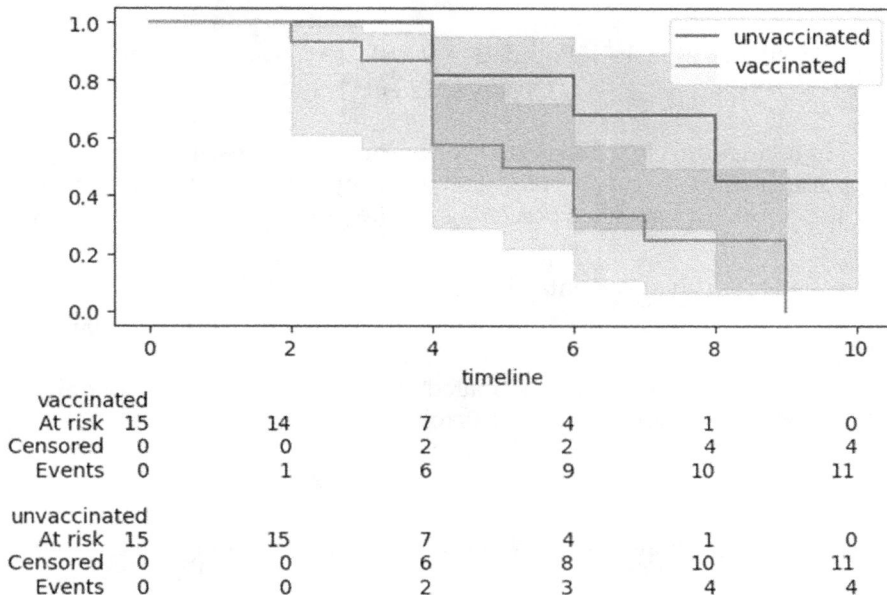

vaccinated						
At risk	15	14	7	4	1	0
Censored	0	0	2	2	4	4
Events	0	1	6	9	10	11
unvaccinated						
At risk	15	15	7	4	1	0
Censored	0	0	6	8	10	11
Events	0	0	2	3	4	4

FIGURE 9.3
Kaplan-Meier curves illustrating survival of patients diagnosed with C-24 over time.

To create the dataset needed for the Kaplan–Meier curve, we must calculate the probability of survival at each time unit t and each treatment group A or B (vaccinated and unvaccinated). Table 9.2 shows event time in years for periods in which there is available data (notice there is no 1 or 2). Furthermore, the mortality count, censored count, population at risk, survival percentage (i.e., mortality percentage), and cumulative survival percentage at each time unit are provided. Here, we can see the value of the censored subjects, which would otherwise be excluded from conventional traditional statistical methods. We might not know when an event occurs for a given censored subject, but their presence in the data remains valuable, in that patients surviving past the study end date remain useful in knowing the population at risk at a given point in time.

Let's look at the notation. First, we must calculate the survival percentage for each time. This is an iterative calculation as the population at risk is conditional events in the preceding time. The calculation is as follows:

$$\text{Survival Percentage}_t^A = \frac{\text{Population at Risk}_t^A - \text{Observed Events}_t^A}{\text{Population at Risk}_t^A}$$

Population-at-risk refers to the remaining population after removing censored data and observed events occurring from prior periods. The notation below t-1 refers to the previous time (or the previous row in Table 9.2).

$$\text{Population at Risk}_t^A = \text{Population at Risk}_{t-1}^A - \text{Censored Count}_{t-1}^A - \text{Observed Events}_{t-1}^A$$

The cumulative survival percentage (or proportion) for each time t is simply the product of the survival percentage (or proportion) for the current time and the cumulative survival percentage of the previous time.

$$\text{Cumulative Survival Percentage}_t^A = \text{Survival Percentage}_t^A \times \text{Cumulative Survival Percentage}_{t-1}^A$$

For example, at year 6 for the vaccinated group, the cumulative survival percentage is 68% (or .68)—calculated as follows:

$$0.68 = .82 \times .83$$

Note that proportions are used here instead of percentages (as a better practice).

TABLE 9.2

Aggregated Patient Data in the Vaccinated and Unvaccinated C-24 Groups to Support the Kaplan–Meier Curve

i	Vaccinated					Unvaccinated				
	O_t^A	q_t^A	n_t^A	Y_t^A	S_t^A	O_t^B	q_t^A	n_t^B	Y_t^B	S_t^B
Time-to-event (Years)	Observed Events (Mortality Count)	Censored	Population at Risk	Survival Percentage for time t	Cumulative Survival Percentage	Observed Events (Mortality Count)	Censored	Population at Risk	Survival Percentage for time t	Cumulative Survival Percentage
0	0	0	15	100%	100%	1	0	15	93%	87%
3	0	4	15	100%	100%	1	1	14	93%	87%
4	2	2	11	82%	82%	4	1	12	67%	58%
5	0	1	7	100%	82%	1	0	7	86%	50%
6	1	1	6	83%	68%	2	0	6	67%	33%
7	0	1	4	100%	68%	1	2	4	75%	25%
8	1	1	3	67%	45%	0	0	1	100%	25%
9	0	0	1	100%	45%	1	0	1	0%	0%
10	0	1	1	100%	45%	0	0	0	0%	0%

The cumulative survival probabilities in Table 9.2 are plotted to form the Kaplan–Meier curves for the two treatment groups (vaccinated and unvaccinated).

The Python *lifelines* library does all these tedious calculations for us to produce a Kaplan–Meier plot for the two treatment groups.

```python
import pandas as pd
from lifelines import KaplanMeierFitter
from lifelines.statistics import logrank_test
from lifelines.plotting import add_at_risk_counts
import matplotlib.pyplot as plt
from lifelines.utils import survival_table_from_events

data = pd.DataFrame({
    'Event Time (Years)': [3, 3, 6, 4, 4, 3, 3, 5, 8, 8,
7, 6, 10, 4, 4, 4, 4, 4, 9, 7, 3, 3, 6, 6, 7, 4, 4, 2, 7,
5],
    'Age': [60, 48, 58, 74, 42, 64, 43, 26, 54, 59, 66,
55, 71, 43, 45, 46, 35, 34, 54, 45, 60, 69, 41, 74, 46,
85, 60, 66, 67, 73],
    'Sex': ['M', 'F', 'F', 'M', 'M', 'M', 'M', 'F', 'M',
'M', 'M', 'F', 'F', 'F', 'M', 'M', 'M', 'F', 'M', 'M',
'U', 'M', 'M', 'F', 'F', 'F', 'M', 'M', 'F', 'M'],
    'Observed Event (Mortality)': [0, 0, 0, 1, 0, 0, 0,
0, 0, 1, 0, 1, 0, 0, 1, 1, 1, 0, 1, 0, 1, 0, 1, 1, 0, 1,
1, 1, 1, 1],
    'Treatment': ['vaccinated', 'vaccinated',
'vaccinated', 'vaccinated', 'vaccinated', 'vaccinated',
'vaccinated', 'vaccinated', 'vaccinated', 'vaccinated',
'vaccinated', 'vaccinated', 'vaccinated', 'vaccinated',
'vaccinated', 'unvaccinated', 'unvaccinated',
'unvaccinated', 'unvaccinated', 'unvaccinated',
'unvaccinated', 'unvaccinated', 'unvaccinated',
'unvaccinated', 'unvaccinated', 'unvaccinated',
'unvaccinated', 'unvaccinated', 'unvaccinated',
'unvaccinated']
})

time_column = 'Event Time (Years)'
event_column = 'Observed Event (Mortality)'

group1_data = data[data['Treatment'] == 'vaccinated']
group2_data = data[data['Treatment'] == 'unvaccinated']

kmf_control = KaplanMeierFitter()

kmf_control.fit(group1_data[time_column], event_
observed=group1_data[event_column], label='unvaccinated')
ax2 = kmf_control.plot()
```

```
kmf_exp = KaplanMeierFitter()
kmf_exp.fit(group2_data[time_column], event_
observed=group2_data[event_column], label='vaccinated')
ax2 = kmf_exp.plot(ax=ax2)

add_at_risk_counts(kmf_exp, kmf_control, ax=ax2)
plt.tight_layout()
```

The dataset used in this code example contains the data in Table 9.1 and is then divided into two groups based on a treatment variable: "vaccinated" and "unvaccinated."

For each group, the code fits the survival data using the KaplanMeierFitter from lifelines, specifying the time and event columns, and labels the respective plots accordingly ('vaccinated' or 'unvaccinated').

The resulting Kaplan–Meier plots for the two groups (vaccinated and unvaccinated) are generated, plotting the estimated survival probabilities over time. The add_at_risk_counts function adds the counts of individuals at risk in each group at various time points on the plots. I like seeing the data table below the plot, but there are many ways to customize the plot output. The reader is encouraged to review the lifelines documentation to tailor the visualization to their needs.

A similar implementation can be achieved using R using the survival library to fit the model, and survminer library to visualize the Kaplan–Meier curve.

```
library(survival)
library(survminer)

data <- data.frame(
  Event_Time_Years = c(3, 3, 6, 4, 4, 3, 3, 5, 8, 8, 7,
6, 10, 4, 4, 4, 4, 4, 9, 7, 3, 3, 6, 6, 7, 4, 4, 2, 7,
5),
  Age = c(60, 48, 58, 74, 42, 64, 43, 26, 54, 59, 66, 55,
71, 43, 45, 46, 35, 34, 54, 45, 60, 69, 41, 74, 46, 85,
60, 66, 67, 73),
  Sex = c('M', 'F', 'F', 'M', 'M', 'M', 'M', 'F', 'M',
'M', 'M', 'F', 'F', 'F', 'M', 'M', 'M', 'F', 'M', 'M',
'U', 'M', 'M', 'F', 'F', 'F', 'M', 'M', 'F', 'M'),
  Observed_Event_Mortality = c(0, 0, 0, 1, 0, 0, 0, 0, 0,
1, 0, 1, 0, 0, 1, 1, 1, 0, 1, 0, 1, 0, 1, 1, 0, 1, 1, 1,
1, 1),
  Treatment = c('vaccinated', 'vaccinated', 'vaccinated',
'vaccinated', 'vaccinated', 'vaccinated', 'vaccinated',
'vaccinated', 'vaccinated', 'vaccinated', 'vaccinated',
'vaccinated', 'vaccinated', 'vaccinated', 'vaccinated',
'unvaccinated', 'unvaccinated', 'unvaccinated',
'unvaccinated', 'unvaccinated', 'unvaccinated',
'unvaccinated', 'unvaccinated', 'unvaccinated',
```

```
'unvaccinated', 'unvaccinated', 'unvaccinated',
'unvaccinated', 'unvaccinated', 'unvaccinated')
)

surv_object <- Surv(data$Event_Time_Years,
data$Observed_Event_Mortality)

km_fit <- survfit(surv_object ~ Treatment, data = data)

plot(km_fit, col = c("blue", "red"), xlab = "Time
(Years)", ylab = "Survival Probability", main = "Kaplan-
Meier Survival Curves by Treatment")

legend("topright", legend = c("Vaccinated",
"Unvaccinated"), col = c("blue", "red"), lty = 1)
```

In this R code, the Surv function creates a survival object that defines the time and event status. The survfit function then calculates Kaplan–Meier survival curves for each treatment group, using the tilde (~) to specify that the curves should be separate for each group.

The Kaplan–Meier curves in Figure 9.3 show that the vaccinated group appears to survive longer than the unvaccinated group. While this is informative as a directional tool, a hypothesis test, such as the log-rank test, will help conduct robust analyses.

Log-Rank Test

Log-rank tests are statistical tools for comparing survival curves between two or more groups. They assess whether there are significant differences in the survival curves (e.g., vaccinated vs. unvaccinated) or if the differences are likely due to chance.

First, we must set up the hypothesis for a log-rank test. Remember the steps for hypothesis testing from Chapter 3?

> **Null Hypothesis H_0:** There is no difference in survival experiences between the vaccinated and unvaccinated groups.

> **Alternate Hypothesis H_a:** There is a difference in survival experiences between the vaccinated and unvaccinated groups.

Note that we are evaluating a difference in survival curves in either direction, so we are conducting a two-tailed test. We'll need to set a significance level before conducting our test, so we'll use the traditional $\alpha = 0.05$ significance level (or 95% confidence level).

Drilling in further, the test statistic for a log-rank test is essentially a chi-squared test designed to work with time data. The test statistic uses observed and expected numbers of events, whereby the sum of squared differences between the observed and expected events at each time is divided by the sum of the variance at each time point. Since the notation in this section is more involved, we'll use some abbreviated field names in this section. The field names and their abbreviations can be found in the header of Table 9.2 and are also redefined in the following.

We'll apply the log-rank test for the unvaccinated group to gain insight into survival differences between the unvaccinated and vaccinated groups. The test statistic can be calculated as follows:

$$\chi^2 \text{ log rank statistic} = \frac{\sum O_i^B - E_i^B}{\sum Var\left(O_i^B - E_i^B\right)}$$

The test statistic follows a chi-square distribution, and therefore, we can obtain a p-value based on this distribution, parameterized by the degrees of freedom (i.e., the number of groups, such as vaccinated and unvaccinated, minus 1). This p-value reflects the probability of observing the obtained differences in events between groups if there's no true difference in survival (i.e., we do not reject the null hypothesis).

I'll note that the statistical notation is a bit squirrely, but stay with me. A worked step-by-step example will follow in plain English.

Let's start with the calculations for the expected counts. The expected event count for a given treatment group (e.g., vaccinated) and time unit t is calculated as the proportion of the population at risk for the treatment group of interest times the total observed cases across both groups. This expected value estimates the count of observed cases that we would expect, assuming no difference between the vaccinated and unvaccinated groups at time t.

For the vaccinated group, expected events for each time t can be calculated as follows:

$$E_t^A = \frac{n_t^A}{n_t^A + n_t^B} \times \left(O_t^A + O_t^B\right)$$

Likewise, for the unvaccinated group, the expected events for each time can be calculated as follows:

$$E_t^B = \frac{n_t^B}{n_t^A + n_t^B} \times \left(O_t^A + O_t^B\right)$$

The variance component helps quantify the variability between the observed and expected events, which in turn contributes to the overall test statistic.

The formula for the variance between the observed and expected values across a given time can be calculated as follows:

$$Var\left(O_t^B - E_t^B\right) = \sum_{t=0} \frac{n_t^A \times n_t^B \times \left(O_t^A + O_t^B\right) \times \left(n_t^A + n_t^B - O_t^A - O_t^B\right)}{\left(n_t^A + n_t^B\right)^2 \left(n_t^A + n_t^B - 1\right)}$$

where

- O_t^A is the number of observed events (deaths) in the vaccinated group at time t.
- O_t^B is the number of observed events in the unvaccinated group at time t.
- E_t^A is the expected number of events in the vaccinated group at time t.
- E_t^B is the expected number of events in the unvaccinated group at time t.
- n_t^A is the total number of patients at risk in the vaccinated group.
- n_t^B is the total number of patients at risk in the unvaccinated group.

Now that we've outlined the conceptual calculations for the log-rank test, let's examine a worked example using the C-24 data scenario. The calculation details are in Table 9.3.

The table lists columns for the expected events for each period and treatment group. For example, the expected number of events for the unvaccinated group in year 4 is approximately 3.13.

$$3.13 = \frac{12}{11 + 12} \times (2 + 4) = \frac{n_t^B}{n_t^A + n_t^B} \times \left(O_t^A + O_t^B\right)$$

The difference between the observed and expected events for each period is summed and squared to produce the numerator of the test statistic (see the column labeled "Observed – Expected" in Table 9.3).

$$3.637 = \sum O_t^B - E_t^B$$

Finally, we calculate the time-specific variance for each period and sum those to obtain the overall variance result of 3.208 (see the "Variance" column in Table 9.3).

$$3.208 = Var\left(O_2 - E_2\right)$$

The final log-rank test statistic therefore is 4.123:

TABLE 9.3

Aggregated Patient Data in the Vaccinated and Unvaccinated C-24 Groups to Support the Log-Rank Test Calculation

	Vaccinated					Unvaccinated					
i	O_t^A	q_t^A	n_t^A	E_t^A	$O_t^A - E_t^A$	O_t^B	q_t^A	n_t^B	E_t^B	$O_t^B - E_t^B$	$\mathrm{Var}(O_t^B - E_t^B)$
Time-to-event	Observed Events	Censored	Population at Risk	Expected Events	Observed-Expected	Observed Events	Censored	Population at Risk	Expected Events	Observed-Expected	Variance
0	0	0	15	0.5	-0.5	1	0	15	0.5	0.5	0.25
3	0	4	15	0.517	-0.517	1	1	14	0.482	0.517	0.250
4	2	2	11	2.870	-0.870	4	1	12	3.13	0.867	1.157
5	0	1	7	0.5	-0.5	1	0	7	0.5	0.5	0.25
6	1	1	6	1.5	-0.5	2	0	6	1.5	0.5	0.614
7	0	1	4	0.5	-0.5	1	2	4	0.5	0.5	0.25
8	1	1	3	0.75	0.25	0	0	1	0.25	-0.25	0.188
9	0	0	1	0.5	-0.5	1	0	1	0.5	0.5	0.25
10	0	1	1	0	0	0	0	0	0	0	0
										3.637	3.208

$$\chi^2 \log \text{rank statistic} = 4.123 = \frac{3.637^2}{3.208}$$

To determine statistical significance, the log-rank test statistic is compared against the chi-square distribution with one degree of freedom (for comparing two groups). Python's lifelines library can perform the log-rank test automatically, along with *p*-values associated with the test statistic.

With that segue, let's look at the Python code to conduct a log-rank test.

```python
import pandas as pd
from lifelines import KaplanMeierFitter
from lifelines.statistics import logrank_test
from lifelines.plotting import add_at_risk_counts
import matplotlib.pyplot as plt
from lifelines.utils import survival_table_from_events

data = pd.DataFrame({
    'Event Time (Years)': [3, 3, 6, 4, 4, 3, 3, 5, 8, 8,
7, 6, 10, 4, 4, 4, 4, 4, 9, 7, 3, 3, 6, 6, 7, 4, 4, 2, 7,
5],
    'Age': [60, 48, 58, 74, 42, 64, 43, 26, 54, 59, 66,
55, 71, 43, 45, 46, 35, 34, 54, 45, 60, 69, 41, 74, 46,
85, 60, 66, 67, 73],
    'Sex': ['M', 'F', 'F', 'M', 'M', 'M', 'M', 'F', 'M',
'M', 'M', 'F', 'F', 'F', 'M', 'M', 'M', 'F', 'M', 'M',
'U', 'M', 'M', 'F', 'F', 'F', 'M', 'M', 'F', 'M'],
    'Observed Event (Mortality)': [0, 0, 0, 1, 0, 0, 0,
0, 0, 1, 0, 1, 0, 0, 1, 1, 1, 0, 1, 0, 1, 0, 1, 1, 0, 1,
1, 1, 1, 1],
    'Treatment': ['vaccinated', 'vaccinated',
'vaccinated', 'vaccinated', 'vaccinated', 'vaccinated',
'vaccinated', 'vaccinated', 'vaccinated', 'vaccinated',
'vaccinated', 'vaccinated', 'vaccinated', 'vaccinated',
'vaccinated', 'unvaccinated', 'unvaccinated',
'unvaccinated', 'unvaccinated', 'unvaccinated',
'unvaccinated', 'unvaccinated', 'unvaccinated',
'unvaccinated', 'unvaccinated', 'unvaccinated',
'unvaccinated', 'unvaccinated', 'unvaccinated',
'unvaccinated']
})

time_column = 'Event Time (Years)'
event_column = 'Observed Event (Mortality)'

group1_data = data[data['Treatment'] == 'vaccinated']
group2_data = data[data['Treatment'] == 'unvaccinated']
```

```
results = logrank_test(group1_data[time_column],
group2_data[time_column],
                        group1_data[event_column],
group2_data[event_column])
print(results.print_summary())
```

The core analysis happens with the `logrank_test()` function from the lifelines library. This test compares the survival experiences of the two groups ('vaccinated' vs. 'unvaccinated') based on their 'days' (time to an event) and 'event' (whether the event occurred or not) columns. Specifically, the log-rank test assesses whether there is a statistically significant difference in the survival distributions between the two groups.

The R code is a bit more compact as it only needs the patient-level data frame (not the group-level aggregations).

```
library(survival)

data <- data.frame(
  Event_Time_Years = c(3, 3, 6, 4, 4, 3, 3, 5, 8, 8, 7,
6, 10, 4, 4, 4, 4, 4, 9, 7, 3, 3, 6, 6, 7, 4, 4, 2, 7,
5),
  Age = c(60, 48, 58, 74, 42, 64, 43, 26, 54, 59, 66, 55,
71, 43, 45, 46, 35, 34, 54, 45, 60, 69, 41, 74, 46, 85,
60, 66, 67, 73),
  Sex = c('M', 'F', 'F', 'M', 'M', 'M', 'M', 'F', 'M',
'M', 'M', 'F', 'F', 'F', 'M', 'M', 'M', 'F', 'M', 'M',
'U', 'M', 'M', 'F', 'F', 'F', 'M', 'M', 'F', 'M'),
  Observed_Event_Mortality = c(0, 0, 0, 1, 0, 0, 0, 0, 0,
1, 0, 1, 0, 0, 1, 1, 1, 0, 1, 0, 1, 0, 1, 1, 0, 1, 1, 1,
1, 1),
  Treatment = c('vaccinated', 'vaccinated', 'vaccinated',
'vaccinated', 'vaccinated', 'vaccinated', 'vaccinated',
'vaccinated', 'vaccinated', 'vaccinated', 'vaccinated',
'vaccinated', 'vaccinated', 'vaccinated', 'vaccinated',
'unvaccinated', 'unvaccinated', 'unvaccinated',
'unvaccinated', 'unvaccinated', 'unvaccinated',
'unvaccinated', 'unvaccinated', 'unvaccinated',
'unvaccinated', 'unvaccinated', 'unvaccinated',
'unvaccinated', 'unvaccinated', 'unvaccinated')
)

log_rank_result <- survdiff(Surv(Event_Time_Years,
Observed_Event_Mortality) ~ Treatment, data = data)

print(log_rank_result)
```

Like the Python implementation, the R code performs a log-rank test to compare the survival experiences of the two treatment groups. The `Surv(Event_Time_Years, Observed_Event_Mortality)` component creates a "survival object" that includes information on the time until an event and whether or not the event occurred (with 1 when the event happened and 0 if it did not). The `~ Treatment` component defines the treatment groups for comparison. The `survdiff` function then conducts the log-rank test, which checks if there is a significant difference between the survival curves of the treatment groups.

The results of this code yield a chi-square test statistic of 4.12 and a p-value of .04. With our significance level of 0.05, we can reject the null hypothesis, which states that there is no difference in survival between the vaccinated and unvaccinated groups in favor of the alternate hypothesis, which states that there is a difference in survival between the vaccinated and unvaccinated groups.

Cox Proportional Hazards

While the log-rank test is helpful in evaluating a single variable, real-world research questions often involve multiple factors. The Cox proportional hazards model, or *Cox regression*, serves this purpose in time-to-event analysis, especially when evaluating multiple factors. It is a tool to help measure the association between predictors (such as treatment and demographics) and the *hazard* of an event. At this point, you are probably annoyed that I haven't defined hazards and hazard ratios, so let's do that now.

Hazards and Hazard Ratios

A hazard refers to the probability of an event occurring within a specific period, given that it has not yet occurred. A higher hazard implies a greater probability of the event happening at any given moment. Hazards are dynamic and can vary over time. They might be higher or lower at different stages compared to the previous time unit, and reflect changes in risk associated with the event.

Hazard ratios, or the ratio of hazards, quantify the relative difference in hazards between groups or conditions within a study. It compares the instantaneous risk of an event occurring at any given time in one group relative to another. The Cox regression model tells us how the hazards of an event change with each unit increase of the predictor. For example, we might be interested in the hazards of the vaccinated group relative to the unvaccinated group but also in controlling for factors such as age and sex. Cox regression will provide an adjusted hazard ratio for this treatment variable while considering the effects of age and sex. Age and sex, too, will have an associated hazards ratio so that we can quantify how hazards might change (linearly) as an individual ages or how risk might differ by the individual's sex.

Hazard ratios are analogous to relative risk in that we evaluate risk (or hazards) for one group relative to another in the form of a ratio. However, hazards differ from relative risk in that relative risk is based on the risk assessed within a fixed time unit. In both cases, the ratios are interpreted similarly, with increased risk (or hazards) for one group relative to another being expressed as a ratio greater than one and decreased risk for one group relative to another being expressed as a ratio less than one.

Cox Regression

When conducting time-to-event analysis in the wild, we typically want to account for multiple risk factors (or predictors). In our C-24 example, it is unlikely that vaccine status is the sole factor that explains survival. Like most diseases, patient characteristics such as age, sex, and disease history are likely to contribute to the survival of those diagnosed with C-24. We've seen that the log-rank test is a helpful tool when evaluating the effect of a single factor (e.g., vaccine or no-vaccine, male or female); however, a more robust approach would be to use the power of regression modeling in the context of survival to provide a better estimate of one factor's association with survival while controlling for other important explanatory variables.

Let's continue with our C-24 example. In addition to vaccine status, we might want to incorporate the age and sex variables available to us in Table 9.1. This way, we can control for potential covariate imbalance (i.e., the

$$
\underbrace{h(t)}_{\text{Hazard}} = \underbrace{h_0(t)}_{\substack{\text{Baseline} \\ \text{Hazard}}} \times \underbrace{e^{\beta_1 X_1 + \beta_2 X_2 + \cdots + \beta_n X_n}}_{\substack{\text{Linear} \\ \text{Combination} \\ \text{of Predictors}}}
$$

unique patient mix) between the two treatment groups by evaluating and controlling for age and sex. We can better understand the vaccine's efficacy by controlling for these factors. Let's review the notation:

We can see from this notation that there are three primary components: (1) the hazard function $h(t)$, (2) the baseline hazard function $h_0(t)$, and (3) the linear combination of predictors $e^{\beta_1 X_1 + \beta_2 X_2}$. The latter component should be familiar to those who read the chapter on regression methods.

We can also express the Cox regression model in log form by applying a natural log to both sides of the equation:

$$ln\big(h(t)\big) = ln\big(h_0(t)\big) \times \beta_1 X_1 + \beta_2 X_2 + \dots + \beta_n X_n$$

We'll start with the hazard function $h(t)$, which serves as the response variable. It represents the probability that an event will occur in a certain time interval, given that the individual has survived up until that point.

Like the regression methods discussed in Chapter 5, $X_1 \dots X_n$ are the covariates (or predictors) while $\beta_1 \dots \beta_n$ are the coefficients associated with each covariate, indicating the magnitude and direction of their impact on the hazard. The component expressed as $e^{\beta_1 X_1 + \beta_2 X_2 + \dots + \beta_n X_n}$ shows that the linear combination of covariates is being exponentiated. Notice, however, that there is no intercept in this equation. In the context of a single predictor, we can think of this as knowing the slope of the line but not the point at which it intersects with the y-axis. The baseline hazard function $h_0(t)$ anchors the linear combination of predictors to produce estimated hazards, in a similar way as an intercept.

Furthermore, the baseline hazard $h_0(t)$ refers to the hazard function associated with an event of interest (such as death and failure) when all explanatory variables or covariates are at zero or in their reference state. It is unique in that the baseline hazard is a function of time t and can dynamically vary across different time intervals. The linear combination of predictors extends the baseline hazard function to account for that added risk based on the unique set of characteristics of the evaluated subjects.

Interpreting Model Output

The model summary of a Cox regression provides helpful information for interpreting how predictor variables are associated with event hazards. It allows us to measure how a one-unit increase in the predictor value is related to the *log* hazards of experiencing the event (e.g., death) at any given time. A Cox regression produces a similar coefficient summary to an OLS or GLM model (Table 9.4).

Since the coefficients from a Cox regression are based on the log hazards, we can exponentiate these values to obtain an adjusted hazard ratio. This is similar to exponentiating the coefficients in a logistic regression to obtain an adjusted odds ratio. Again, given that the model is fit based on the values of all covariates, the hazards ratio, in this case, is an adjusted ratio that controls for the effects of the remaining variables.

The Cox regression output also includes a 95% confidence interval, a z-score, and a p-value for each predictor in the model. You guessed it, we are

TABLE 9.4

Summary Output of the Predictor Variables from a Cox Regression

	Coef (Log Hazard Ratio)	se(coef)	coef lower 95%	coef upper 95%	z	p
Age	0.05	0.03	0	0.1	1.91	0.06
Sex_M	0.71	0.63	−0.52	1.93	1.13	0.26
Treatment_ vaccinated	−1.11	0.6	−2.29	0.08	−1.83	0.07

hypothesis testing again! In the context of Cox regression, we are interested in determining if there is a statistically significant association between the predictor (or covariate) and the hazards of an event. We can't prove a statistically significant association, so we must state in the null hypothesis that there is no association (i.e., the status quo) and gather evidence to reject the null hypothesis in favor of the alternate hypothesis with some predetermined confidence level. The hypothesis statement can be expressed as follows:

> **Null Hypothesis H_0 :** The null hypothesis states that there is no association between the covariate and the hazard of the event occurring, which we can represent as

$$H_0 : \beta = 0$$

> **Alternative Hypothesis H_a :** There is a non-zero association between the covariate and the hazard of the event. It's represented as

$$H_a : \beta \neq 0$$

Notice that the alternate hypothesis states that there is a non-zero association. This means that we are conducting a two-tail test, whereby the null hypothesis will be rejected if the p-value derived from the test statistic is lower than the predetermined significance level (alpha = .05 in this case).

A hazard ratio of 1 means no effect, a hazard ratio greater than 1 implies a higher hazard, and a hazard ratio less than 1 suggests a lower hazard compared to a reference level or for a unit change in a predictor. The hazard ratio indicates the magnitude and direction of a predictor's association with the hazard.

Looking at Table 9.5, containing the exponentiated coefficients (or adjusted hazard ratios), we can see that when controlling for age and sex, vaccine treatment is no longer a statistically significant variable (within our predetermined confidence level). If I were conducting this analysis, however, I would not discount these results altogether. The odds ratio of .33 indicates that there is a 66% lower hazard of death for vaccinated patients compared to the

TABLE 9.5

Summary Output of the Predictor Variables from a Cox Regression, with Exponentiated Coefficients and 95% Confidence Intervals

	exp(coef) (Hazard Ratio)	exp(coef) lower 95%	exp(coef) upper 95%	z	p
Age	1.05	1	1.1	1.91	0.06
Sex_M	2.03	0.59	6.92	1.13	0.26
Treatment_vaccinated	0.33	0.1	1.08	−1.83	0.07

unvaccinated group, and the p-value is relatively low considering the number of observations. With these results, one might decide to conduct a more extensive study or include additional explanatory variables (such as the days since the vaccine)—all while being cautious about conducting analysis until we get the desired answer (*p*-value hacking). Remember that significance testing requires us to set an arbitrary threshold, and nothing magical happens at the .05 alpha level. From this study, we can report our findings (the association is not statistically at the set alpha level), even if they are not what we were hoping for, and recommend further analysis to assess the vaccine's efficacy.

Assumptions

In every statistical analysis, we must check the model assumptions. Some of the assumptions in Cox regression are consistent with those in OLS and GLM models. First, outcomes should be independent. That is, the outcome (e.g., survival time) of one patient should not depend on (or be associated with) the survival time of another.

Additionally, the relationship between continuous predictors and the log of the hazard rate (i.e., outcome) should be linear. This assumption ensures that the association between predictors and the hazard rate remains constant and does not exhibit nonlinear relationships that could bias the model's estimates.

Unique to the Cox regression model are the assumptions of proportional hazards and non-informative censoring. The proportional hazards assumption states that hazards associated with different levels of predictors must remain proportional over time. This means the hazard ratios between any two groups remain constant throughout the study period. Recall that hazards may increase and decrease over time; however, the assumption here is that the difference in hazards between two groups (e.g., male and female, or treatment and no-treatment) will remain consistent (proportional) over time. If the risk ratio of a vaccine is .33 (66% lower hazard of death), we assume that regardless of time, the risk difference remains the same.

The last assumption involves *non-informative censoring*, whereby data censoring should be unrelated or independent of the outcome of interest. In other words, the probability of being censored should not be influenced by the likelihood of experiencing the event being studied.

Now that we've trudged through the details of Cox regression, we can move on to your favorite part, the Python code. Again, using the lifelines library, we can fit a Cox regression, adding risk factors for age and sex in addition to the treatment (vaccinated or unvaccinated).

```python
import pandas as pd
from lifelines import CoxPHFitter
data = pd.DataFrame({
    'Event Time (Years)': [3, 3, 6, 4, 4, 3, 3, 5, 8, 8,
7, 6, 10, 4, 4, 4, 4, 4, 9, 7, 3, 3, 6, 6, 7, 4, 4, 2, 7,
5],
    'Age': [60, 48, 58, 74, 42, 64, 43, 26, 54, 59, 66,
55, 71, 43, 45, 46, 35, 34, 54, 45, 60, 69, 41, 74, 46,
85, 60, 66, 67, 73],
    'Sex': ['M', 'F', 'F', 'M', 'M', 'M', 'M', 'F', 'M',
'M', 'M', 'F', 'F', 'F', 'M', 'M', 'M', 'F', 'M', 'M',
'U', 'M', 'M', 'F', 'F', 'F', 'M', 'M', 'F', 'M'],
    'Observed Event (Mortality)': [0, 0, 0, 1, 0, 0, 0,
0, 0, 1, 0, 1, 0, 0, 1, 1, 0, 1, 0, 1, 0, 1, 1, 0, 1,
1, 1, 1, 1],
    'Treatment': ['vaccinated', 'vaccinated',
'vaccinated', 'vaccinated', 'vaccinated', 'vaccinated',
'vaccinated', 'vaccinated', 'vaccinated', 'vaccinated',
'vaccinated', 'vaccinated', 'vaccinated', 'vaccinated',
'vaccinated', 'unvaccinated', 'unvaccinated',
'unvaccinated', 'unvaccinated', 'unvaccinated',
'unvaccinated', 'unvaccinated', 'unvaccinated',
'unvaccinated', 'unvaccinated', 'unvaccinated',
'unvaccinated', 'unvaccinated', 'unvaccinated',
'unvaccinated']
})

data = pd.get_dummies(data, columns=['Sex', 'Treatment'],
drop_first=True)
print(data.columns)

cph = CoxPHFitter()
cph.fit(data, duration_col='Event Time (Years)', event_
col='Observed Event (Mortality)', formula="Age + Sex_M +
Treatment_vaccinated")

cph.print_summary()
```

In the above code, categorical variables like 'Sex' and 'Treatment' are encoded into binary indicators using one-hot encoding to make them usable for the CoxPH model. The CoxPH model is fit using the `CoxPHFitter()` function from the lifelines library, considering the effect of age, male sex (`'Sex_M'`), and being in the vaccinated treatment group (`'Treatment_vaccinated'`) on the time to the event. The code then prints out a summary of the fitted CoxPH model, which includes statistical information about the coefficients (or effects) of age, male sex, and being in the vaccinated group, along with other relevant statistics like p-values and confidence intervals.

Using R, we can again use the survival package. We'll also use the `dummy_cols` function from `fastDummies` package to create dummy (or "one-hot-encoded") variables for the categorical values. This can also be done with base R, but it's a helpful library to keep the code nice and clean.

```
library(survival)
library(fastDummies)

data <- data.frame(
  Event_Time_Years = c(3, 3, 6, 4, 4, 3, 3, 5, 8, 8, 7,
  6, 10, 4, 4, 4, 4, 4, 9, 7, 3, 3, 6, 6, 7, 4, 4, 2, 7,
  5),
  Age = c(60, 48, 58, 74, 42, 64, 43, 26, 54, 59, 66, 55,
  71, 43, 45, 46, 35, 34, 54, 45, 60, 69, 41, 74, 46, 85,
  60, 66, 67, 73),
  Sex = c('M', 'F', 'F', 'M', 'M', 'M', 'M', 'F', 'M',
  'M', 'M', 'F', 'F', 'F', 'M', 'M', 'M', 'F', 'M', 'M',
  'U', 'M', 'M', 'F', 'F', 'F', 'M', 'M', 'F', 'M'),
  Observed_Event_Mortality = c(0, 0, 0, 1, 0, 0, 0, 0, 0,
  1, 0, 1, 0, 0, 1, 1, 1, 0, 1, 0, 1, 0, 1, 1, 0, 1, 1, 1,
  1, 1),
  Treatment = c('vaccinated', 'vaccinated', 'vaccinated',
  'vaccinated', 'vaccinated', 'vaccinated', 'vaccinated',
  'vaccinated', 'vaccinated', 'vaccinated', 'vaccinated',
  'vaccinated', 'vaccinated', 'vaccinated', 'vaccinated',
  'unvaccinated', 'unvaccinated', 'unvaccinated',
  'unvaccinated', 'unvaccinated', 'unvaccinated',
  'unvaccinated', 'unvaccinated', 'unvaccinated',
  'unvaccinated', 'unvaccinated', 'unvaccinated',
  'unvaccinated', 'unvaccinated', 'unvaccinated')
)

data <- dummy_cols(data, select_columns = c("Sex",
"Treatment"), remove_first_dummy = FALSE)

cox_model <- coxph(Surv(Event_Time_Years, Observed_Event_
Mortality) ~ Age + Sex_M + Treatment_vaccinated, data =
data)

summary(cox_model)
```

The code is fairly straightforward. Setting `remove_first_dummy` = `FALSE` ensures that all categories, including the reference category, are kept in the model. The `Surv` function creates a survival object (as we have seen with the log-rank test). The `coxph` function fits the Cox proportional hazards model using the age and sex predictors.

The results of this model have been provided in Tables 9.4 and 9.5.

Summary

In this chapter, three methods were discussed to evaluate and model time-to-event data.

The first method discussed was the Kaplan–Meier curve, which creates visual survival curves, estimating event probabilities over time and accommodating censored data along the way. This non-parametric technique presents survival probabilities across time periods and further allows groups to be compared across time.

The Log Rank Test was also introduced as a complement to the Kaplan–Meier curve which allows us to statistically compare survival curves between groups in the form of a hypothesis test. Finally, the section on Cox Proportional Hazards introduces a statistical model designed for time-to-event analysis, particularly in understanding various factors' impact on hazard rates. Hazards represent the likelihood of an event occurring within a specified timeframe, while hazard ratios compare these risks between different groups or conditions.

Additional Resources

Klein, J. P., & Moeschberger, M. L. (2003). *Survival Analysis: Techniques for Censored and Truncated Data* (2nd ed.). Springer-Verlag New York.

Index

Pages in *italics* refer to figures and pages in **bold** refer to tables.

For Product Safety Concerns and Information please contact our EU
representative GPSR@taylorandfrancis.com
Taylor & Francis Verlag GmbH, Kaufingerstraße 24, 80331 München, Germany